(MIS)DIAGNOSED

(MIS)DIAGNOSED

HOW BIAS DISTORTS OUR PERCEPTION OF MENTAL HEALTH

JONATHAN FOILES

Belt Publishing

Printed in the United States of America
First edition 2021
1 2 3 4 5 6 7 8 9

ISBN: 978-1-948742-99-3

Belt Publishing
5322 Fleet Avenue
Cleveland, Ohio 44105
www.beltpublishing.com

Cover art by David Wilson
Book design by Meredith Pangrace

For Edmond

"Psychotherapy takes place in the overlap of two areas of playing, that of the patient and that of the therapist. Psychotherapy has to do with two people playing together. The corollary of this is that where playing is not possible then the work done by the therapist is directed towards bringing the patient from a state of not being able to play into a state of being able to play."

—Donald Winnicott, "Playing: A Theoretical Statement"

TABLE OF CONTENTS

INTRODUCTION

A young woman sits across from me, a shock of bleach blond hair obscuring her face. Her gaze is focused on the tissue she is twisting in her hands. Bits flake off like snow and fall on the floor in front of my desk. She is here for an intake interview, beginning the process of unraveling her life story to get the help she has realized she needs. Her mother is already one of our patients; she is down the hall speaking with her psychiatrist.

Madeleine has told me that she is concerned about her depression, and she relates a number of symptoms that meet criteria for the diagnosis: persistent depressed mood, poor sleep, poor appetite, loss of interest in activities that used to interest her, lack of energy. She tells me that she has thought about killing herself. She also mentions that her entire family has discussed mass suicide, a disclosure that chills me as I try to calmly assess the seriousness of the threat. Her father overdosed on heroin just last week and was brought back with naloxone. It's happened so often that she's lost count. Hopelessness is the water in which her family swims.

Before I proceed on to the myriad of other questions her public aid insurance forces me to ask her prior to beginning treatment, I check through a mental list of other symptoms to make sure I'm on the right track.

"Do you ever have times when you feel the opposite of depressed, like you could do anything and don't even need to sleep?"

Her tear-brightened eyes jump up to meet mine. "Well, actually, yeah, sometimes I'll stay up all night and clean and clean the house even though it doesn't need it. I might sleep an hour or two or I might go a few days without sleep, but I actually feel pretty great."

"Do you have any issues with anger or irritability?"

Shame descending, she replies, "Well, um, yeah, I do tend to yell quite a bit and cuss out my family. I mean, I've never hit them or anything, but I might throw things, punch the wall, stuff like that."

"During those times, do you do things you wouldn't really think of doing otherwise or things that are considered to be pretty risky?"

She stares at me uncomfortably. "Um, well, this is confidential, right?"

I assure her that it is.

"Well, anyway, I have tried cocaine when I feel like that, just to make the feeling last, you know? But I haven't really told anyone that before."

With a few more questions, I am reasonably confident that bipolar disorder better fits her experience. Setting aside the keyboard I have been using to type up my clinical impressions, I lean forward to give her the news.

"Based on what we've talked about so far, I think that you have bipolar disorder. It is serious, but it is also very treatable. I'm really glad that you came in and decided to ask for help. Do you have any questions I can answer right now?"

For the first time, a smile cracks across her small face. "I just thought I was crazy this whole time. I honestly just feel relieved to know there's a name for all of that, you know?"

———————

Later in that same office, I sit across from one of my therapy clients, a young man named Michael. Someone else has already done his intake, and he arrives with a diagnosis: schizophrenia. Not that I needed to be told. While the word "schizophrenia" most often conjures up images of a person seeing or hearing things that aren't there, or conjuring fantastic narratives that aren't true (known as positive symptoms), the disorder also includes what we call negative symptoms—things that take away from a person's normal functioning. There's an interior hollowness, a depletion of one's energy, an inability to feel much of anything. Most people with schizophrenia will say those symptoms are the hardest part, and the medications that we have right now do little to help address them.

Michael reports experiencing much of this, and like many millennials, he has turned to the internet to help him understand his symptoms. This has led him into the wastelands of YouTube and its algorithm, and he tells me what he saw.

"I've been watching videos of other people who are diagnosed with schizophrenia, older people. They were saying that life has been hell for them, and it just gets worse and worse. A lot of them said that they want to die."

He is both right and not right, as I try to explain to him. If schizophrenia is detected early, as his was, the outcomes are much better than if it is allowed to progress untreated. Since it is usually a disease that strikes in young adulthood, precisely when most of us feel that we're invincible anyway and have no need to see a doctor, this is often easier said than done. However, the severity of the episodes Michael has experienced to date is concerning, and his psychiatrist has yet to find an antipsychotic that hits the middle ground of blunting his symptoms without erasing his core identity. I try to explain all of this as gently as I can, but I can feel the tightrope underneath my feet.

"So what you're saying is that you can't really be sure, but they could be right? I just . . . I don't want to end up like that. I can't."

I end up doing something that I wouldn't do now, and that is to try to match his stories of endless suffering with those of other people with schizophrenia who have managed to thrive. From the perspective of the present, I realize that instead of allowing both of us to sit with his feelings, I grew uncomfortable—scared even—and acted out of my fears. But at the time, I did what I thought would help.

Together, we watch a TED Talk by Elyn Saks, an accomplished USC law professor who has also been diagnosed with schizophrenia. I can tell he is unimpressed, but he is kind and humors me. At the conclusion of our session, I check and he assures me that he has no plans to try to kill himself.

Michael won't tell me for some time, but he will continue to watch those YouTube videos. He grows more distressed as he imagines what his future holds, sees all the ways it might be constricted. When one of the videos mentions a way to kill yourself that is supposed to be relatively quick and pain-free, he will think about it. Months after our conversation, after several other sessions, he will try it when his family and I least expect it. But his story doesn't end there; he will be hospitalized then and a few other times, and somewhere along the way he will find the right combination of medications.

They will help restore him to himself, and he will begin to allow himself to dream. He will start to relate to the idea of "schizophrenia" in a different way.

What does it mean to be diagnosed with a "mental illness"? If you ask most people, they would probably tell you that mental illnesses are caused by a chemical imbalance in the brain. This view, first promulgated in the late 1950s and early 1960s, has now been thoroughly debunked by professionals, but it continues to persist in the absence of any concrete evidence.[1] At the time the chemical imbalance theory was first proposed, modern psychiatry was still in its infancy and struggling to legitimize itself as a medical discipline in the face of much skepticism from other branches of medicine, that were more obviously based upon biology. It didn't help that prior to the invention of psychotropic medication the primary tools of psychiatry were often brutal: electroshock therapy, insulin comas, lobotomies. The idea that mental illnesses were due to our brains failing to keep certain neurotransmitters in proper balance placed psychiatrists on the same level as other medical professionals, as psychiatrists had long desired. Diseases of the mind were no different than diseases of the body.

That may be how it started, but the real staying power of the chemical imbalance theory is thanks to the pharmaceutical industry. The idea that depression in particular is caused by low levels of a neurotransmitter called serotonin was a problem to which drug companies had a readily available answer: selective serotonin reuptake inhibitors, or SSRIs, by far the most commonly prescribed class of drugs for depression.

An early television ad for Zoloft depicts a sad-looking blob lying underneath its own personal rain cloud, impervious to the call of a songbird nearby. The narrator solemnly intones the symptoms of depression. As the music shifts into a major key, a graphic of "Nerve A" and "Nerve B" appears, with neurotransmitters moving between them. The narrator says, "While the cause is unknown, depression may be related to an imbalance of natural chemicals between nerve cells in the brain. Prescription Zoloft works to correct this imbalance. You just shouldn't have to feel this way anymore." The blob, suddenly happy and in the sunshine, is now able to listen to the songbird as it flies through the air. The tagline at the end reads "Zoloft: When you know more about what's wrong, you can help make it right."[2]

Even if it's not scientifically accurate, perhaps the chemical imbalance theory is a useful corrective to lingering societal stigma, an assurance that the one suffering is not making it all up. While I have not used the theory to explain symptoms to my clients, I rarely correct them when I've heard them espouse it, hoping they find it helpful in some way. It turns out, though, that I am wrong: a 2014 paper found that when patients were given a bogus test to prove their depression was caused by a chemical imbalance, it did not reduce their self-blame, worsened their expectations for improving, and caused them to be disposed more favorably toward psychopharmacology rather than psychotherapy. (Another win for the drug companies, I suppose.)[3]

Today, pharmaceutical companies make relatively modest claims about the causes of depression and the mechanisms of cure. The website for the newer antidepressant Trintellix, for example, says, "Experts believe that depression (MDD) results when certain chemicals in the brain are out of balance. These chemicals, called neurotransmitters, send messages from one brain cell to another by acting at specific receptors. Although it's not fully understood, Trintellix is thought to work by enhancing the activity of a neurotransmitter called serotonin in the brain by blocking serotonin reuptake. It also has activities on some of the receptors for this brain chemical. The link between this information and the therapeutic benefit is not known." This hardly reads like a ringing endorsement, but it is relatively transparent about the current state of our knowledge.

The shifts within pharmaceutical advertising reflect an ambiguity that persists regarding the etiology of mental illness. If your doctor suspects you may have diabetes, there is a simple way to find out: draw some blood, measure the blood sugar in the sample, and compare it to the range for healthy adults in order to determine whether or not it meets the criteria for the diagnosis. We currently have no way to measure the presence of serotonin or any other neurotransmitter in a patient who presents with symptoms of depression. In addition to being incorrect, the chemical imbalance theory has never had a test to legitimate its claims. Yet it has had staying power because it neatly fits our current age's obsession with medicalizing all forms of human suffering.

A diagnosis of depression, or any other mental illness for that matter, is made purely based on observation and patient self-report. If I suspect you have depression like I first thought with Madeleine, I will ask you similar questions about the state of your mood, how well you have been sleeping and eating, if you have maintained contact with your support network, if your job or school responsibilities have suffered, if you are able to stay interested in your activities. If these symptoms have lasted for longer than two weeks and a sufficient number of them are met, then you officially have major depression.

While some continue to hope that neuroscience will finally address many lingering questions about the depths of the human brain, we are still quite far from that possibility. The popular discourse regarding mental illness only makes sense to us given the circumstances of our understanding and what we think counts as both mental health and mental suffering. It is a product of what the philosopher Arnold Davidson calls a "psychiatric style of reasoning," which only arose around the 1870s.[4]

Mental "diseases," whether ones we continue to utilize like depression or those that have been relegated to the dust heap like hysteria, are unlike other prior conceptions of illness in that they are disorders of function rather than of a diseased organ or other somatic component. That is, they are diagnosed based upon what one *does*, and while early psychiatry held out the hope that these could be proven to be the result of some physical change or disorder, such evidence has proved elusive. This deviation from traditional notions of health and disorder served, in Davidson's words, "to create entire new species of diseased individuals, and to radically alter our conceptions of ourselves." We had to first think about ourselves in a certain way before the idea of mental illness made any sense. This does not mean that previous societies have not had similar notions, of course, but the discourse we use to explain how someone might suffer from an invisible but pernicious malady is a product of a host of other developments that has far removed us from prior conceptions of the causes of mental illness, such as a punishment from god(s) or oppression from evil spirits or witches.

Between 1870 and 1905, the developing discipline of psychiatry found itself caught between neurology and psychology. Thinkers of equal stature debated whether mental suffering was due to physical differences in brain structure or something more ephemeral but no less real. To fully illustrate these tensions, we can look at the evolving understanding of homosexuality. In order to adequately describe why homosexuality should be considered a disease, psychiatry first had to create an idea of the sexual instinct, a pattern of behavior that was "normal" and that thus defined what was abnormal. This was not at all a given prior to the psychiatric era, when men who had sex with men were criminals and punished for the "crime" of sodomy rather than for *being* homosexuals. Such a concept did not yet exist. The advent of the sexual instinct and its goal-oriented behavior, heterosexual reproduction, gave rise to a class of people who did not share this aim, not as a function of a particular act but based upon their core sense of self. This created homosexuality, alongside other such "deviations" as masochism, sadomasochism, and bestiality. Psychiatrists initially focused on what physical defects could cause men to sexually desire other men. (Lesbians often went unnoticed and were far less the subject of psychiatric concern.) One leading French psychiatrist conjectured that homosexuality arose from a malformed male uterus. As their knowledge of anatomy progressed and they discovered that men who had sex with men had no appreciable physical differences from other men, psychiatry then contended that it must be due to malformations in the brain itself. The fact that autopsies failed to confirm such a hypothesis did not dissuade its adherents. The cause was still physical; it just became more difficult to trace and, in that regard, more impervious to critique.

No responsible medical professional now regards homosexuality as a sign of mental disorder. So what changed?

Our concept of human sexuality as a whole did. The sexual instinct became uncoupled from being solely a means of procreation thanks to larger social shifts that took place in the 1960s. As our view of sex began to expand, theoretical room was made for alternative expressions of sexuality. Alongside this, we also began to do a better job of listening to gay and lesbian voices who contradicted the vagaries of our prior theory with their lived experience. They did not seem to be suffering from their sexuality, so the categorization of homosexuality-as-disease no longer fit.

The historical progress of mental disorders still widely used and seen to be genuine in a way homosexuality no longer is does not look that different. The Greek Hippocrates and the Roman Galen both believed that melancholia was caused by an imbalance of black bile, one of the four humors, or bodily fluids, that cause illness and suffering when not existing in the proper ratio. Here again, mental illness only made sense as the product of some somatic complaint. Kraepelin, one of the founders of modern psychiatry, theorized in the late nineteenth century that the various forms of depression were neurological in origin, and although they could be triggered by external events, they were largely independent of them. He had no way of proving this, however, and autopsies failed to confirm his theory. Decades later, the chemical imbalance theory came into vogue. Somatic imbalance to neurological malfunctioning to invisible chemical malady: the progression is the same.

There are differences too, of course. Depression is a condition that impacts many, but few would argue that it is an essential part of one's personhood in the same way as one's sexuality. Many find ways to flourish *despite* it but not *through* it. Even more important, psychotherapy can help alleviate the experience of depression, while it can do nothing to change one's sexuality. We have strong data to assert the former and none to support the latter. That does not mean that our idea of depression is necessarily more correct than the earlier theories of a humoral imbalance or neurological deficit, however. Like most other mental illnesses, depression is a phenomenon in search of an etiology. As Supreme Court Justice Potter Stewart once famously said, "I know it when I see it," yet knowing where it comes from is something else entirely.

The elusive search for a cause for depression, or any other mental illness for that matter, can obscure the important fact that we do know several factors with which it is correlated. That is, we can't definitively point to a specific trigger for a depressive episode, but we do know characteristics that people with depression typically share. Children who are bullied or witness one parent physically abusing another parent are far more likely to become depressed, for instance.[5] In adults, the risk of depression increases with most serious illnesses. There appear to be some genetic factors at play too, but even these aren't necessarily as clear-cut as they might seem. If you grow up in a household saturated by trauma or lacking basic necessities due to your socioeconomic status, it makes sense that depression would seem to be grafted onto the family tree. You don't need to consult someone's genetic material; just take a look around their house and their neighborhood.

Things don't change that radically even if we consider mental illnesses that upon first glance appear far more random. Risk factors for schizophrenia include prenatal maternal stress, maternal malnutrition, childhood trauma of all sorts, the death of a parent, being bullied, social isolation, discrimination due to one's housing status, family dysfunction, unemployment, and poor housing conditions. Genetics deserves a place here too, but what genes get expressed depend upon many of these variables.

If we are serious about reducing mental illness, this gives us a lot to work with. Growing up in a safe environment with adequate resources and without being discriminated against provides a strong buffer against mental anguish. Yet we almost never frame mental illness in terms of the conditions of our society, preferring instead to focus upon the individual and, perhaps, their immediate family. This differs from how we talk about other illnesses that impact the body. Most laypeople could probably not explain the mutations that cause lung cancer or the fluctuations in blood sugar that cause diabetes, yet we know we can insulate ourselves from these illnesses to a not-insignificant degree by not smoking and eating right. Even here, though, the focus remains tightly confined to the individual. Anti-smoking campaigns have erected billboards and signs in low-income neighborhoods for decades, often coexisting alongside major polluters and other sources of carcinogens that never seem to merit the same level of attention as a pack of cigarettes.

In most instances, we can't point to a definitive cause for a mental illness. When they do occur, they often happen alongside other societal factors that increase human misery. Given this reality, some have suggested that we give up on the idea of mental illness altogether. The anti-psychiatry movement began in the 1960s alongside other liberatory movements, contending that diagnoses were social constructs used by those in power to proscribe behavior and punish outliers, no more scientific or useful than earlier claims about demons or witches.

I am sympathetic to this view, but I cannot quite go there. I have met more than a few clients like Madeleine for whom a diagnosis serves as a lifeline, a reassurance that what they are experiencing remains in the realm of the human. Whether or not the diagnosis names something "real" is often beside the point. Esmé Weijun Wang writes in *The Collected Schizophrenias* of her search to find the proper diagnosis, suspecting that the diagnosis bipolar disorder did not fully encapsulate her experiences. After many conversations with her psychiatrist, she received a diagnosis of schizoaffective disorder and writes of its impact: "A diagnosis is comforting because it provides a framework—a community, a lineage—and, if luck is afoot, a treatment or cure. A diagnosis says that I am crazy, but in a particular way."[6] It can be powerful to have your craziness named, to be assured that this too is human, however terrifying that prospect.

Not everyone feels comfortable in their newly assigned community, however. As Michael illustrates, to be placed into a category of the suffering can also be terrifying. Often it is both at once. In the cases of both Madeleine and Michael, though, what really matters is not the diagnosis itself. A diagnosis, after all, is just a series of words created by medical professionals to better communicate with one another. Rather than listing all of Michael's symptoms each time I talked with his psychiatrist or other professionals, I can tell them he has schizophrenia, which clusters his symptoms together and suggests a course of action. It is everything that happens after that point that can make a diagnosis sting. If Michael feels that his diagnosis changes how his family sees him or causes his psychiatrist to dismiss his preferences and experiences, what was once a single, rather odd word comes to stand in for a bundle of pain and hurt.

We continue to live in the era of psychiatry—antidepressants are among the most prescribed drugs in the United States. Yet the inner workings of the mind remain a mystery to us. It is fairly straightforward to describe what a fully functioning kidney looks like and how to know when things go awry, far less so when the object of concern is the mind. The diagnoses we use to establish the line between normal and abnormal functioning shift and change with time. There have been diagnoses that are all the rage in a certain era only to fall by the wayside as our understanding of ourselves has shifted. Sometimes it is not the winds of change that erase a diagnosis but those who have been saddled with it and instead advocate that their behavior falls within the confines of the normal.

Diagnoses rarely disappear entirely. Their fossilized remains lurk within the pages of the *Diagnostic and Statistical Manual of Mental Disorders*—a thick tome better known as the *DSM*, now in its fifth edition, which is put out by the American Psychiatric Association. In this book, I intend to embark upon an excavation, plumbing contemporary diagnoses that trouble me to unearth other concepts long forgotten whose logic nevertheless remains intact in our current formulations.

My aim for this archaeological project is twofold. Contrary to what many think, diagnoses are helpful but by no means necessary for the work of psychotherapy. They are crucial if one is to prescribe medication or bill an insurance provider, of course, but they don't play nearly as large of a role in two people talking to one another. When a client comes to me and tells me that they have been diagnosed with bipolar disorder, depression, or the like, I file it away in my head as necessary data. However, that categorization is far less interesting or meaningful to me than exploring what gives their life purpose and how they could better live into their values. To paraphrase the British psychoanalyst Donald Winnicott, the business of therapy is really just two people playing together. I have found that the fear of diagnosis, what it might mean to be labeled as "depressed" or "anxious," much less "psychotic," prevents many people from consulting a therapist when they need help. A label that isn't all that useful to my work serves as an impediment to those in need.

Perhaps it's time to rethink the utility of those labels, or at least how we relate to them. Once I know the person sitting in front of me has schizophrenia, the focus becomes fixed on treating their hallucinations and delusions, on helping them best integrate into society. We thus exempt ourselves from considering everything that came before they entered our office. What if it was possible to both acknowledge their suffering while also condemning the injustices and inequalities that have helped lead them here? That is the task that I have set for myself in the following pages.

CHAPTER 1
PATHOLOGIZING PROTEST

When I worked in community health, I wore a variety of hats for my patients. I talked to them about their mental illness, of course, but I also helped them look for jobs and housing, discussed how they could share their experiences with other medical professionals, explained the slow process to attain disability benefits, and worked on many other things that I was not taught in school but picked up piecemeal along the way. Social workers take pride in being flexible, in doing what it takes to help those in need.

Thus, I wasn't surprised to be explaining to a longtime patient of mine named Al that he shouldn't "act crazy" (his words) at his upcoming disability hearing. Al had been assigned the diagnosis of schizoaffective disorder by his psychiatrist long before I started seeing him. Schizoaffective disorder, a branch of the schizophrenia tree, means that a person experiences the symptoms one would usually associate with schizophrenia (hallucinations, delusions) but also experiences the symptoms of depression and/or mania in the absence of such psychotic symptoms. It's somewhat of a bridge diagnosis between major depression or bipolar disorder and the psychotic disorders.

Al was hoping that this diagnosis, along with some physical maladies, would suffice to convince the judge to award him disability benefits. A few decades prior, he had been a hairdresser, but racism had forced him to the suburbs to find work. When the shop where he worked closed, he found that his other options had dried up too. Occasionally, I would mention the variety of part-time jobs that existed in the neighborhood, but Al had grown up there and would often remind me that his long-deceased father had earned $15 per hour working in the factories that used to be in the neighborhood—before they fled to the suburbs along with the white people. He did not want to earn less than that years later. It was hard to argue with such logic.

Al did not have to "act crazy" to get approved for disability; he let his voluminous records do the talking. Our sessions consisted of reminiscing about his childhood, processing the racism both overt and covert that he had experienced throughout his lifetime, and discussing the news of the day. I believed that he did truly suffer mentally; he had very little contact with people other than me, didn't trust people, and seemed to hear and see things that weren't there. I used to see a lot of patients like Al. There was also Marvin, who believed he had inherited an ability to see and talk to spirits; Teddy, who claimed to be tormented by the sound of babies crying; Eric, whose outbursts of intense anger caused him shame and guilt in the aftermath. All had mental health symptoms that plagued them and shaped their interactions with others. All were also Black men. The strands of their stories were so infused with suffering that it was difficult to separate their symptoms from their history. Was Al depressed because he often self-isolated, or did he self-isolate because the only people he knew around him had chronic substance abuse issues? Was Marvin paranoid because some neurotransmitters in his brain were out of balance, or because he had been beaten by police upon multiple occasions in the past? How much of Eric's anger was due to the fact that he had very few friends left because so many of them had been murdered? All had ended up with diagnoses of severe mental illness along the schizophrenia spectrum, yet there was clearly more at work in each case.

There are a variety of diagnoses that can include psychotic symptoms, both perceiving things that aren't there (hallucinations) and believing things that are not true (delusions). People with bipolar disorder can experience hallucinations when in a manic state. If one is depressed and also experiences psychotic symptoms, the diagnosis often given is major depression with the psychosis modifier added on. Aside from mental illness, there are a variety of things that can cause someone to hallucinate, memorably catalogued by the neurologist Oliver Sacks in his book *Hallucinations*: lack of sleep, migraines, certain forms of dementia, brain injuries, sensory deprivation (as in solitary confinement), and so forth. So if a client says that they perceive things that aren't there or that have some outlandish beliefs, there are several diagnoses that could accurately include those experiences. Schizophrenia is usually thought to represent the far reaches of this continuum, the most serious of serious mental illnesses.

Black Americans—and Black males, in particular—are far more likely to be diagnosed with schizophrenia as compared with patients of other races, despite the fact that all ethnicities experience the disorder at the same rate.[1] This doesn't just stop at diagnosis, though. Black people are also less likely to receive mental health services in the first place,[2] and the care that they receive is often poorer. One study of a community mental health center's prescribing patterns found that whites were six times more likely to receive a second-generation antipsychotic medication—the contemporary treatment of choice for schizophrenia—while Black people were prescribed older drugs with riskier side effects.[3] Black people are often subject to more coercive treatments, such as shots received on a regular basis instead of an oral medication.[4] These depot medications can be great for people who struggle to remember to take their medicine, but they can also take away the element of choice from clients and become a tool of social coercion.

Contrary to what you may think, this is, by and large, a Western problem. It is well-documented but underreported that outcomes are actually better for people with schizophrenia in less-developed countries. Beginning in the 1960s, researchers from across the world began meeting together to determine whether or not schizophrenia was a cultural construct or a malady present across cultures. They ended up deciding in favor of the latter option, but upon their trips to the various member countries of the International Pilot Study of Schizophrenia, they noticed a recurring phenomenon. Two American psychiatrists visiting Nigeria, John Strauss and Will Carpenter, were initially alarmed to see a woman whom we would diagnose with schizophrenia chained to a post in the yard of a local traditional healer. Once they recovered from their shock, however, they realized something important: despite the admittedly poor conditions in which she was kept, the woman did not experience social isolation from her fellow villagers; she engaged in regular conversations with passersby who were happy to stop and chat with her.[5] To be clear, we should not chain up those with mental illness, yet when we do it in the West, we don't put the people with schizophrenia in the middle of the community. Instead, we lock them away from everyone else.

People with schizophrenia in the United States are often highly marginalized, and those on the margins are far more likely to be diagnosed with the illness. Few of us encounter people with schizophrenia on a regular basis, or at least few of us realize it when we do. This has something to do with its prevalence rate: the National Institute of Mental Health reports between 0.25 and 0.64 percent of Americans have schizophrenia compared to 7.1 percent of adults who have experienced a depressive episode. This may seem like a paltry figure, but the prevalence rate for having red hair is between 1 and 2 percent, and most if not all of us can recall past interactions with redheads.

The history of schizophrenia in America is far more complex than we may assume. To illustrate how the diagnosis of schizophrenia has evolved over time, the researcher and psychiatrist Jonathan Metzl examined the patient charts from a now-shuttered state hospital in Michigan. For most of the first half of the twentieth century, schizophrenia was seen as the result of an overworked mind. The type of patient who ended up with the diagnosis looked far different than those I would meet in community mental health a few generations later. Instead of being a time bomb set in place by one's genetics, it was a possibility that could develop over the course of one's life if one had a certain personality configuration. The prototypical patient was dreamy, childlike, and unconnected to reality. It was a serious illness, yes, but it was also thought to include notable benefits such as an artistic temperament and increased sensitivity to others and their needs. Treatment often took the form of occupational therapy, exercise, and social activities. These patients were still mistreated, of course, and not all treatment was as gentle, yet people with schizophrenia were by and large not seen as a threat to the rest of humanity.

The 1948 film *The Snake Pit* reflects this version of schizophrenia. In the film, Olivia de Havilland plays Virginia Cunningham, an institutionalized woman with schizophrenia. The film does not shy away from the realities of asylums—the title refers to the level of care reserved for the lowest-functioning individuals who are placed in padded cells and abandoned—yet care is taken to depict Cunningham's life before her institutionalization, focusing in particular on her marriage. The film ends with de Havilland's character recovering and leaving the asylum behind.

Modern films that deal with schizophrenia continue to be interested in depicting their (almost always white) protagonists overcoming their illness and thriving. In *The Fisher King* (1991), Parry, played by Robin Williams, helps Jack, played by Jeff Bridges, atone for the sins of his shock jock past and conveniently reawakens from his illness once his mythic quest is completed. Perhaps the most notable recent film to depict schizophrenia, *A Beautiful Mind* (2001), does not depict the protagonist as completely cured at the end, but his symptoms do not prevent him from winning the Nobel Prize.

America began to change in the 1960s as the civil rights movement spread across the country, and the concept of schizophrenia evolved alongside these societal shifts. As the nonviolent rhetoric of leaders like Martin Luther King Jr. gave way to the more militant approach of groups like the Black Panthers, mental health became another means of policing racial boundaries. For example, the second edition of the *DSM* (1968) expanded the definition of schizophrenia, and for the first time, hostile and aggressive behavior were included as symptoms of the paranoid subtype. That same year, Drs. Walter Bromberg and Franck Simon published an article in the *Archives of General Psychiatry* titled "The 'Protest' Psychosis: A Special Type of Reactive Psychosis."[6] In the article, Bromberg and Simon describe a new form of psychosis, ostensibly based on what they were seeing in their incarcerated patients, which was "influenced by social pressures (the Civil Rights Movement), dips into religious doctrine (the Black Musslim [sic] Group), is guided in content by African subcultural ideologies and is colored by a denial of Caucasian values and hostility thereto. This protest psychosis among prisoners is virtually a repudiation of 'white civilization.'" Symptoms included the usual hallucinations and delusions but also encompassed antisocial behavior, interest in pan-Africanism or Islam, and attempts to develop an "anti-white" language. Bromberg and Simon theorized that the disorder arose when Black men became overwhelmed by their largely unconscious feelings of hatred toward whites and retreated toward "an African ideology" in order to assuage their guilt over the crimes they committed against the white race.

The racism is obvious, yet Bromberg and Simon were not outliers. Prominent ads for antipsychotics displayed crazed-looking Black mental patients, while other academic articles warned that Black men could develop psychotic symptoms as a result of participating in sit-ins or become delusional due to believing their civil rights had been violated. Perceived Black militancy became not just dangerous to the white world but a sign of insidious illness. Black people literally disappeared into their "hatred" and fear of whites and became mentally ill. Such a move both allowed whites to disregard anything that Black Americans might say, since it was evidence of their shattered thinking, and institutionalize those who did speak up or revolt. Label someone's thoughts as delusional and you ensure that neither you nor anyone else have to take them seriously. While the racism is less overt, it's hard not to think of Al and others like him here as well: labeling them along the schizophrenia spectrum allows us, however implicitly, to sweep up all their other experiences under the mantle of their illness.

Schizophrenia has been politicized elsewhere as well as a tool to punish those who question the status quo. In the former Soviet Union, Dr. Andrei Vladimirovich Snezhnevsky, the foremost psychiatrist in the country for decades, believed that the diagnostic confines of schizophrenia were too narrow. He instead proposed that the severity of the illness could be plotted along a continuum. At one end lay the severe cases, those who are obviously mentally ill, and at the other end was "sluggish schizophrenia." Sluggish schizophrenia could be almost anything, including minor behavioral issues, and need not include hallucinations or delusions. It preserved the stigma of schizophrenia without any of the actual symptoms and served as a handy diagnostic tool to discredit dissidents and punish them with years of "treatment." As Dr. Walter Reich points out, it is probable that some of these diagnoses were not made in bad faith; rather, dissent did seem strange to most Soviet citizens, and the weakened concept of sluggish schizophrenia gave them a tool to provide an easy explanation for how someone could act so without casting a critical eye at their own society.[7] Something similar is at play in claiming that Black protest is a sign of mental distress rather than a reminder of the legacy of white supremacy. Condemnation of Soviet psychiatry was widespread at the time, but few have turned a similarly critical eye to our own practices.

The sort of mental institutions that used to house large numbers of patients for years at a time have all but disappeared. The institutionalized population of people with mental illness has shifted from asylums, which at least theoretically offered treatment to reduce suffering, to jails and prisons that house Black and Brown people in ever-increasing numbers. One estimate attributes 7 percent of the overall growth in the prison population from 1980 to 2000 to the deinstitutionalization of people with severe mental illness, landing an additional 40,000 to 72,000 people in jail or prison.[8] Mental illness is far overrepresented in the inmates housed in such institutions; according to the American Psychological Association, 64 percent of those in jail, 54 percent of those in state prisons, and 45 percent of those in federal prisons have a mental illness,[9] compared to a baseline rate of about 20 percent in the general population. Conditions associated with the modern prison industrial complex—including overcrowding, pervasive threats of violence, and the overuse of solitary confinement—are practically designed to further inflame the symptoms of mental illness. Any "treatment" incarcerated individuals receive is often aimed at blunting their symptoms to make them docile and compliant, not to restore them to health. Returning citizens often go back to chronically underdeveloped neighborhoods with few options available to receive mental health treatment, ensuring the cycle of mass incarceration and the criminalization of serious mental illness continues.

In thinking through the ways that schizophrenia has been used to silence the resistance of Black people against an often irrational society, I am reminded of another diagnosis once used to explain the supposedly inexplicable actions of Black Americans. Samuel Cartwright was a physician in the American

South during the nineteenth century who sought to answer a question that perplexed him and many of his peers: what caused enslaved people to seek to run away? Cartwright believed that behind this phenomenon lay a heretofore undiscovered mental illness that he labeled "drapetomania" in 1851, a portmanteau combining the Greek words for "runaway slave" and "mad or crazy." While this "mental illness" had been theorized in the Southern judicial system since at least the 1820s, Cartwright was the first to propose both a diagnosis and a cure.[10] Enslaved persons did not seek to run away because of the brutality of the slavery economy but because they were mentally ill, just as a century later Black people protested Jim Crow not to fight for their rights but because they were psychotic.

Drapetomania was not only a Southern construct. It remained an object of general fascination across America that enslaved people could seek to throw off their shackles and run for freedom, a point usually made with reference to the supposedly pleasant conditions in which enslaved people were held. According to Cartwright, this was precisely the problem. Drapetomania arose because conditions were allowed to get too comfortable across the plantations of the South. As he wrote, "On Mason and Dixon's line, two classes of persons were apt to lose their negroes: those who made themselves too familiar with them, treating them as equals, and making little or no distinction in regard to color; and, on the other hand, those who treated them cruelly, denied them the common necessaries of life, neglected to protect them against the abuses of others, or frightened them by a blustering manner of approach, when about to punish them for misdemeanors. Before the negroes run away, unless they are frightened or panic-struck, they become sulky and dissatisfied. The cause of this sulkiness and dissatisfaction should be inquired into and removed, or they are apt to run away or fall into the negro consumption."[11] Cartwright proposed a golden mean for enslavers, not becoming too nice and thus failing to remind enslaved people of their status while also not brutalizing them to the point where they would consider revolt.

Is it fair to compare schizophrenia with a racist construct long-ago consigned to history's wastebasket? While there is no question that schizophrenia names some people's experiences in a way drapetomania never could, there are some similarities that should give us pause. As noted earlier, most of the factors correlated with schizophrenia result from structural inequality and oppression, which are the modified forms of that which kept Black people enslaved for centuries. It is also a documented fact that members of minority communities, particularly Black people, are far more likely to be diagnosed with schizophrenia as well as to be treated with drastic, often brutal methods. It is possible for an illness to also be a means of social control (such as AIDS), and that is often the case with schizophrenia.

To say that one's thoughts and beliefs fly in the face of logic is a profound claim to make. I have met people in the grips of delusional systems that defy common sense, yet these beliefs often paper over profound hurt and loss. And it's entirely possible to get it wrong: the clinic where I used to work had a day program for people with serious mental illness, offering group therapy and other outlets for social connection to people who were often profoundly isolated. One young woman who attended that group displayed her suffering vividly, regularly scratching at the air and yelling profanities at attackers only she could see. It was not apparent to anyone that she had graduated from a notable art school and received glowing write-ups of her paintings before she started hearing voices. Saying that someone is seeing things that aren't there or believes things that aren't true is an invitation to dive deeper in order to help them, not an excuse to write them off and bury them underneath powerful medications.

We know that people with schizophrenia have the best outcomes when they are able to maintain their lives in their community, receiving the help and support they need while not being removed from where they come from.[12] Mass institutionalization and mass incarceration shatter these bonds, stealing Black lives from their communities and subjecting them to the ever-increasing carceral state. Unfortunately, far too many neighborhoods and cities lack the sort of infrastructure to enable anyone, with or without mental illness, to lead a thriving existence. Al had never left his neighborhood, but it had long ago left him. In my practice, I've met many others like Al who need help that their communities can't—or won't—provide.

If drapetomania and schizophrenia both reflect how the majority population sees the lives of minority populations, what label does it assign to its own problems? There is a modern malady seemingly tailored for the excesses of consumer capitalism, but to fully understand its roots, we have to look farther back to a disorder once thought to be so common and so unique to our country and its practices that it acquired the nickname "Americanitis."

CHAPTER 2
AMERICANITIS

When I left community mental health to join a private practice in the Hyde Park neighborhood of Chicago, my work changed in ways both large and small. I was freer to practice in a way I wanted while no longer constrained by a large hospital system. Being able to set my own schedule was certainly a luxury. The type of patients I saw changed too, of course. However, I have found that one of the unavoidable aspects of being human is suffering, so the difference was not as pronounced as one might think.

Due to my proximity to the University of Chicago, I began to see a number of students. While I deeply enjoyed this, I couldn't help but notice the ways in which their undergraduate experience differed from mine. For example, one of my patients, Philip, was a first-year undergraduate from the West Coast. His parents both immigrated to the United States from their South Asian country in pursuit of better employment opportunities. By the time Philip, an only child, was born, they were well-established in their careers and firmly ensconced in the upper middle class. They paid to send Philip to an elite private high school, and he excelled there. He was especially gifted in and interested in public policy, which made the University of Chicago his top choice. His stellar

transcript made him one of the 7 percent or so of applicants the university selected.

Before I met Philip, I spoke to his mother. She had found my contact information online and reached out to see if I would be able to help her son. Since moving to Chicago he'd had a difficult time, making few friends and struggling in his classes. The University of Chicago is quite a studious place (its unofficial nickname for some time was "where fun goes to die"), so he was not lost to partying or the other sort of bacchanalian pursuits one might assume. Nevertheless, he was not doing well, so I agreed to begin seeing him.

I found Philip to be immensely bright and a pleasure to talk to, but it was clear that something profound had changed between the time he graduated from high school and entered college. His high school grades were excellent, but now he found himself on academic probation. He admitted this to me sheepishly, noting that it was the first time he had experienced any real struggle in school. As we discussed his academic history, it became clear that he had experienced some issues with attention and concentration for a while but was able to develop compensatory behaviors that still allowed him to excel. Once he had entered college, though, those behaviors had dissipated almost overnight.

The quality of work expected from students can often rise quite quickly in the transition into higher education; I still remember receiving a C, my first, on a response paper I submitted at the beginning of my college career. This was certainly a factor for Philip as well, but there seemed to be more at work here. When he sat down to do his homework, he explained to me, he was often surrounded by his phone, steadily chirping as friends interacted with him across a variety

of social media apps, an open browser tab with YouTube videos, another with a series on Netflix, and usually a tablet containing some other combination of digital distractions. These had an almost narcotic-like effect upon him; he would describe opening an app or website only to find he had wasted several hours on it, in the same manner as other clients of mine would describe substance binges.

It wasn't just Philip who reported this. I have seen a number of students, usually in the first year of their undergraduate program, who describe the same phenomenon to me. These behaviors often end in a diagnosis of attention deficit hyperactivity disorder and prescriptions of powerful stimulant medications. And it wasn't just my patients reporting such issues. My peers did too. I still recall sitting around a table with my social work classmates, eating lunch and passing time between periods, when several of them who were a few years younger than me reported using stimulants such as Ritalin or Adderall in undergrad to help them complete papers or study all night for tests.

While I attended a Big Ten university for undergrad, I led a pretty tame existence, so I assumed I just missed out on this aspect of the college experience. I became curious, though, and when I began to research the usage of stimulants, the class of drugs that includes Ritalin and other medications used to treat ADHD, I found out that the prevalence of abuse had expanded rapidly in just a few years. Between 2006 and 2011, stimulant abuse among the general population of adults increased by 67 percent, and emergency room visits grew by 156 percent. Estimates of how many undergraduate students have abused stimulants vary wildly but tend to average around 17 percent. Most people who take these medications without a prescription have the same motivation as my patients like Philip, to do well on their academic work, rather than attempting to get "high." And abuse is not limited to undergraduates; roughly the same percentage of graduate students abuse the medications as well. This is not just an American problem—findings from Germany, Switzerland, and Iceland, among others, echo the statistics found in the United States.[1]

To have so many stimulants floating around out there, of course, means that there are enough diagnoses of ADHD to merit those prescriptions. Between 1997 and 1998, roughly 6 percent of American children were diagnosed with ADHD; from 2015 to 2016, that number was over 10 percent.[2] This roughly correlates with my own experience. While I remember a few classmates who struggled with attention or concentration, they were never a significant portion of any given classroom I was in as a child.

What exactly is going on here? Have our genes changed that rapidly, or are other factors at work?

Just like we saw with schizophrenia, there are profound racial disparities in both who gets diagnosed and who gets treatment, but here the roles are reversed. White children are more likely to be diagnosed with ADHD, and when diagnosed, they are more likely to receive prescriptions for stimulants.[3] The *DSM-5* altered the diagnostic criteria in 2013, no longer requiring it to first manifest in childhood in order to be diagnosed in adults, which opened the door to a potential wave of new diagnoses and new prescriptions. Since this happened, I have witnessed an increase in adult clients who report genuine concerns about their ability to maintain their concentration while doing work.

Experts contend that ADHD is not a uniquely American diagnosis and that the rise in diagnoses is the direct result of increasing sensitivity to the disorder aided by decades of research.[4] This may very well be true, but it's hard to miss the ways in which ADHD reflects many of the peculiar values of our society. Many of the students I see are expected to produce an extraordinary amount of work in just a few weeks. They often feel like there aren't enough hours in the day to do the work, and often it seems like they're right. One of my patients recently remarked to me that she thought she was doing well in terms of her sleep because she was averaging six hours a night; most of the other people she knew slept for four or five hours.

These bad habits continue once students graduate and join the workforce. We are the only major developed country that does not mandate any paid time off for its workers; 23 percent of Americans receive no paid time off and 22 percent receive no paid holidays.[5] Even when we receive paid time off, we use it at a rate far below that of other countries with comparable economies. While thinking through this, I remembered speaking with a friend a few years ago who had just landed a job at a start-up. The work world he described to me seemed far removed from anything I had experienced: a fridge stocked with beer for office happy hours, plentiful snacks and free food, a dress code that was almost nonexistent. He and his coworkers were also able to set their own schedules and take as much vacation time off as they wanted. I asked him how they got any work done. It was simple, he explained: everyone was afraid of being outworked and thus being seen as expendable, so they all put in long hours and rarely tapped into that "unlimited" vacation time. I came to see such "perks" as bribes to maintain an unhealthy work-life balance rather than actual benefits.

One study produced by Marriott Hotels found that American business travelers multitasked more than their peers from other countries.[6] Multitasking has increased across generations: millennials are more prone to multitasking than members of Generation X, who are more likely to multitask than baby boomers.[7] The science on multitasking is quite clear: the more that one multitasks, the more diffuse one's attention grows and the harder it is to switch between activities. As someone who took pride in writing papers in college while watching movies and talking to my roommate, I did not want to believe this, but the data is clear.

Americans as a whole are also increasingly sleeping less. The number of American adults saying they sleep less than seven hours a night, the minimum recommended amount, has risen from 30.9 percent in 2010 to 35.6 percent in 2018.[8] The people who are sleeping the least are often those who most need to be well rested: healthcare workers, members of the military, and transportation workers. Among the ruling class, some take a sort of pride in how little sleep they get. Trump often claimed to get by on only four hours per night, and Barack Obama was known to sleep around five hours per night while president. This is not exactly reassuring when you consider how much sleeplessness can impact one's decision-making and general clarity of mind.

Americans thus work more than their peers in other countries, try to accomplish more tasks while working, and get less rest in between workdays. While the diagnostic criteria of ADHD may be equally met by those in other societies, the peculiarity that is American late capitalism encourages us to attempt to do more with less time and then labels the result of such behavior a mental illness. Often, this only occurs if you are part of the privileged class, restricting any such treatments to those with means. The rise in wellness culture (mindfulness, yoga, etc.) may seem like a counterbalance to such excesses, yet if we stop to think about it, do we really believe that massive conglomerations are offering mindfulness classes or yoga instructors out of pure beneficence? Rather than being seen as ends in and of themselves, such practices are often promoted as productivity boosters, aids to increasing one's workflow. "Wellness" is too often a thin sugarcoating applied to the bitter pill late capitalism has prescribed us.

This is not the future that we were promised. In 1930, John Maynard Keynes predicted that in the twenty-first century, we would work fifteen hours a week and enjoy a five-day weekend.[9] A 1965 Senate subcommittee was somewhat more modest in its estimate, believing that by 2000, automation and the rise of computers would reduce the average workweek to twenty hours. In the advanced world of flying cars and robot nannies of *The Jetsons,* George Jetson only had to work three days a week for three-hour shifts. Herbert Marcuse believed that advances in society would dramatically alter the relationship between work and labor, writing in his *Eros and Civilization* (1955): "relieved from the requirements of domination, the quantitative reduction in labor time and energy leads to a qualitative change in the human existence: the free rather than the labor time determines its contents."

These predictions turned out to be half-right: productivity has indeed increased dramatically over the past forty years. An analysis of total economic productivity data from the Bureau of Labor Statistics reveals that productivity has risen by almost 70 percent from 1979 to 2018, yet wages have only risen about 15 percent.[10] Rather than our increased output leading to increased leisure, we have made those at the top far richer than most of us can imagine while the rest of us are scraping to get by despite being a part of one of the most advanced economies in the world. The COVID-19 pandemic only accelerated these changes, making the likes of Jeff Bezos far richer while around a third of Americans could not afford their rent or mortgage.

Ours is not the first age to see rapid shifts in the workforce, of course. In the era following the Civil War, America began to rapidly industrialize, both as a sign of the times and to make up for the labor lost from formerly enslaved persons. Bereft of forced labor under the enslaver's lash, the massive plantations of the South became far less productive, and the already advancing industrial sectors in the North cemented their dominance over the nation's economy. This led to a wave of citizens living in close proximity to one another in cities and settlements rather than being spread across the country in isolated homesteads. As these shifts cemented themselves, a new disease seemed to be plaguing the newly minted managerial class.

At that time, the dominant theory regarding the operation of the nervous system believed individuals were powered by a finite store of energy capable of being depleted. The neurologist S. Weir Mitchell hypothesized that this was happening far more frequently due to the rapid shifts in society: "the cruel competition for the dollar, the new and exacting habits of business, the racing speed that the telegraph and railway have introduced into commercial life, the new value that great fortunes have come to possess as means towards social advancement, and the overeducation and overstraining of our young people, have brought about some great and growing evils, is what is now beginning to be distinctly felt."[11] Different era, same concerns. Another neurologist, George Beard, coined a term for this condition in 1869: neurasthenia.

Neurasthenia did not strike all equally, however. The disorder was thought to be the result of an overworked mind, and in late nineteenth- and early twentieth-century America, not everyone was thought to have the mental capacities for such strain: people of color, predictably, but also Catholics whose devotion to the Pope robbed them of the capacity for critical thinking. To qualify as a neurasthenic, one had to be a WASP of a certain class. It was thought to impact both men and women equally but for differing reasons. Men were overworked due to the larger societal shift away from manual labor and toward what we would now call white-collar jobs, and women were overtaxed by shifting gender standards that opened up more social opportunities and, with them, new stressors.

Neurasthenia was more of a social phenomenon rather than a strict diagnosis, but proposed symptoms included indigestion, fatigue, muscle pain, infertility, impotence, depression, and irrationality. Really, though, if you thought you had it, you probably did—as long as you were white and upper-class. A list of figures diagnosed with neurasthenia reads like a who's who of the American upper class near the turn of the century: William James (who nicknamed the disease "Americanitis"), Max Weber, Jane Addams, and Theodore Roosevelt, among others.

Just as the cause was different for both men and women, so was the cure. Men who contracted neurasthenia were told to get away from their urban offices and reconnect with nature.

They were often sent out West to ride horses, sleep outside, and do other such approximations of the cowboy lifestyle. Theodore Roosevelt exemplifies this approach. While the popular image of him is of a virile outdoorsman and hunter, he was born in Manhattan into a wealthy family and was a sickly child. At twenty-five, he went to the Dakota Territory to hunt bison and, invigorated by the West, bought a cattle ranch. Five years later, he would fight in the Spanish-American War alongside his Rough Riders, finally banishing all trace of his former self.

Women, on the other hand, were prescribed a rest cure to help restore their energy. They were forced to stay in bed for weeks at a time, spoon-fed their meals, and massaged to prevent their muscles from atrophying. They were not allowed to read or move themselves at all, and unsurprisingly, they usually ended up gaining a fair amount of weight from the experience.

Charlotte Perkins Gilman was subjected to such a rest cure by the aforementioned S. Weir Mitchell, and she wrote her famous short story, "The Yellow Wallpaper" in response. Despite renting an estate for the summer, the unnamed narrator is confined to the upstairs nursery by her husband, also a doctor, in order to treat her "slight hysterical tendency." Feeling unmoored by the lack of virtually all outside stimuli and kept confined like a prisoner, the narrator slowly loses her mind, believing that a figure of a woman is formed from shapes in patterns in the titular wallpaper and, upon the conclusion of her "treatment," tells her shocked husband that she is in fact that woman and has finally escaped her two-dimensional confinement.

"The Yellow Wallpaper" helps illustrate the regressive social politics behind the neurasthenia pandemic. After the Civil War, America began to modernize, and its citizens began to further congregate in urban environments and work jobs far removed from the manual labor that until then was the norm and came with its own set of gender and social expectations. Although the rights of women at that time appear virtually nonexistent compared to the present, the fact that American women now could socialize together in larger numbers was another significant shift. No longer were they isolated on family farms or small rural homesteads. The "epidemic" of neurasthenia represents an attempt to move back into an idealized past, to a time when men wrested their bounty from the earth and women were largely isolated in the home to care for them and their children. Neurasthenia was a simultaneous revolt against the perceived feminization of men engaged in white-collar work and the masculinization of women allowed to congregate together.

While Weir, Beard, and other progenitors of the diagnosis were undeniably conservative in their approach, they did not seek to overturn the advances of industrialization. Rather, they instituted "cures" that nodded to these shifting social conventions while allowing the changes instituted by capitalism to continue unabated. Men were encouraged not to abandon their jobs but to make room for more rugged masculine pursuits as well, thus erasing the possibility that gender equality could come about through urbanization and a shifting economy. Women, on the other hand, were reinscribed into their domestic roles and reminded of the power patriarchy held over them by the so-called resting cure. While most did not go mad like Gilman's unnamed protagonist, their confinement continued beyond the cure. Neurasthenia, then, acknowledged the social transitions caused by industrial capitalism and proposed a panacea for treating them, thus ensuring workers would continue in their roles and the system would continue to develop.

This did not go for all workers, of course. Those whose labor did not involve a sufficient degree of intellectual activity were thought to be immune to neurasthenia. The majority of Americans at the time still worked in manual labor sectors regardless of race, and the diagnosis was strictly reserved for those who were white, well-to-do, and Protestant. It was this select group that was to be the prime beneficiary of the late industrial period, and despite the fact that it could cause this novel disorder, they were ultimately the ones whose futures were secured by the same factors that made them suffer.

Today, few think that each person has a finite well of energy that is in danger of being depleted. We do speak that way, however, when it comes to our attention. We complain that certain television shows and books fail to capture our attention, we strive to give our children adequate attention when they need it the most, and we complain that we cannot focus at the end of a long and trying day. Just as industrial capitalism taxed one's mental reserves, so does our late capitalism strive to capture our attention. This happens so frequently that we often fail to notice it; I cannot view any webpage these days, from the highbrow to the low, without seeing ads sprinkled throughout that reflect my own tastes and preferences as preserved on my computer for advertisers. I watched such ads shift and mutate as I left college and became a working professional, got married, had children. In the midst of the COVID-19 pandemic, they shifted from the usual consumer goods to offer me N95 masks and hand sanitizer.

Since we live such saturated lives, it is no wonder that we find our attention often lacking these days. Instead of this being a side effect of our increasingly busy lives, though, what if that is the point? We work more than our peers in other countries, take fewer breaks, allow ourselves less time for rest, and try to do a multitude of things at once. When this process becomes overwhelming, we label it as a disease, both in us and in our children. The fact that these patterns are observable in such young lives should give us serious pause as we consider whether the way we live is working or not, but instead we medicate or treat our shattered attention instead of asking what precisely broke it in the first place.

And not all count, of course. It is still white children who most often get diagnosed with the disorder and, once diagnosed, receive the recommended treatment. One must work hard enough to have one's attention fractured, just like one's job had to be mentally straining enough to merit the diagnosis of neurasthenia. It should come as no surprise that those who are left outside the bounds of ADHD are precisely those who are least served by late capitalism. Class plays a role too, of course; even those patients I see who don't come from wealthy backgrounds have access to a range of services through the university that most could only dream of.

That is not to say that Black children who struggle with attention and concentration fail to receive any notice. There is a diagnosis often reserved for Black children who present difficulties in the classroom: oppositional defiant disorder (ODD). Symptoms of ODD include a pervasive pattern of an angry or irritable mood, argumentative tendencies, defiant behavior, and vindictiveness. Research has suggested that when presenting with the same symptoms, white children are more likely to get diagnosed with ADHD while both Black and Latinx children are more likely to receive a diagnosis of

ODD.[12] Think about the radical difference between being told you are having trouble in school because of a problem with your attention versus attributing it to being defiant and disruptive. One diagnosis assures the student that it is not their fault; the other asserts that it most certainly is. A diagnosis of ODD colors not just how a student views themselves but how teachers and other administrators view them. The increasing presence of police and accompanying harsh disciplinary measures in our schools has created a school-to-prison pipeline, and giving a child a diagnosis of ODD allows them to pass to the front of that line.

ODD is just another variation on the protest psychosis, this time for children and teens rather than adults. Philip did not quite fit this pattern, of course, but if his academic troubles had begun earlier, or if his parents had remained stuck in low-income jobs, chances are I never would have seen him in my office; an academic institution like the University of Chicago would have been rendered far out of reach for him before he even began to think about what he might do with his life.

Let us consider again those medications frequently prescribed to those with ADHD that have become so prone to misuse. Adderall, one of the go-to drugs for treatment of the disorder, is a mix of four amphetamine salts. Chemically, it is almost identical to methamphetamine. Most other medications used to treat the disorder act in a similar manner even if their chemical composition is slightly different. Methamphetamine was first widely used during World War II when both the Axis and Allied powers relied upon it to keep their troops awake and alert. Until the early 1960s, you could buy methamphetamine over the counter as an inhalant. It was used to treat narcolepsy, asthma, and, most popularly, as a weight-loss tool. As data about the potential for abuse grew, methamphetamine use began to be regulated in 1970. Efforts to discourage and criminalize the use and manufacture of meth grew in the 1980s, not coincidentally as usage began to grow among men who have sex with men. At present, meth use is most often associated with poor rural whites and people of color as illustrated by depictions in popular media such as *Breaking Bad* and *Winter's Bone*.

Most college students would never dream of smoking meth to help them write a paper overnight or concentrate better upon the task at hand, yet the only substantial difference between meth and other stimulants is the method of ingestion and the dosage. If it is smoked, it's for "white trash." If it is put into pill form and picked up at a CVS or Walgreens, it becomes a needed prescription medication. The shifting stigma associated with stimulants is a legacy of the so-called War on Drugs begun under President Nixon and continued with aplomb by every succeeding political regime, Democrat or Republican. Almost all drugs that we now consider taboo, not to mention illegal, were once easy to obtain. It was only when they became associated with minorities (Mexicans with marijuana, Chinese for opium, and Black people for heroin) that they became prohibited and coded as socially undesirable.

It can seem that there are two different Americas, one largely white and privileged that is granted access to the best our economy has to offer and the help they need when they need it, and another, mostly Black and Brown, left to get by on the margins. Such a construct is understandable but not all that helpful, for it can make it sound like we're dealing with two different realities. What we really have is two different ways of talking about the same phenomena. When privileged children (who become privileged adults) struggle in the classroom, we see these struggles as the product of an underlying illness and adjust our strategies to suit their needs: more time on tests, extra instruction, and the like. When children of color (and the adults they become) struggle in a similar manner, we see the problem as a part of who they are and subject them to disciplinary measures to shape their behavior to better fit our manner of doing things.

Neurasthenia and ADHD are disorders of privilege, by and large relegated to the ruling classes who have the most access to services and treatment. The ways in which we've defined such diagnoses sharply delineates what is considered suffering and what is behavior to be managed. This extends all the way to the manner in which various drugs are made licit when they come from a prescriber's pad but illegal when they come from the streets. The same dynamic is at play in states, including my own Illinois, that have legalized marijuana. The criminalization of marijuana devastated Black and Brown communities for generations, and prisons are still full of people convicted of marijuana-related crimes. Drug use occurs at the same rate across races and ethnicities, but what is considered a harmless bit of fun for white people becomes criminal when engaged in by minorities. Now that the tides have turned toward decriminalization, it is overwhelmingly white businesspeople who are reaping the benefits. Here in Chicago, almost all of the dispensaries that have opened are located on the (majority white) North Side. As of this writing, no people of color have received a license to open a dispensary, and the communities most ravaged by the War on Drugs are shut out of the newly legal marketplace.

The question is ultimately about whose suffering counts, who gets to have their difficulties adjusting to a new reality acknowledged and, hopefully, treated. For centuries, this has been almost the sole provenance of the mostly white upper and middle classes in America. Whether a behavior is regarded as a legitimate struggle or improper resistance often has far less to do with the actual actions of a person than with how we describe those actions, both to ourselves and to others.

Race is not the only category with such a substantial diagnostic divide. There are also profound differences in diagnoses between genders, even diagnoses that are thought to occur in roughly equal proportions. This problem has been with us since the beginning of psychiatry, starting with the phenomenon that helped launch Sigmund Freud's career. The name has changed, but little else has

CHAPTER 3
ON THE BORDERLINES

For many years, I ran a weekly therapy group aimed at clients who had trouble regulating their emotions and interacting with others. The group utilized an approach called Dialectical Behavior Theory (DBT). As I would explain to the group members, things like learning how to anticipate and respond to your emotions or how to best ask for what you need from others aren't hardwired in us but are taught to us by our parents and other influential figures. If this doesn't happen, you may not know how to navigate such situations through no fault of your own. Although the clients who filtered in and out of the group came from a variety of different backgrounds, many had a shared diagnosis: borderline personality disorder (BPD), the condition that DBT was created to treat.

During one session, a newly diagnosed member brought in a bright yellow book called *F*ck Feelings*, a self-help book written by the Harvard-educated psychiatrist Michael I. Bennett and his daughter, comedian Sarah Bennett. "Do you know what this says about us?" she asked the group, indignant. I didn't, but I had an inkling. I began to cringe before she started reading.

She found the definition of borderline personality disorder and began: "These are the people, usually women, who lonely, crazy-prone single guys often find irresistible. . . . Their dates (and friends and family) are always walking on eggshells, which makes sense when you're dealing with someone who treats each thought and feeling as empirical truth; i.e., 'I am attracted to that guy' quickly becomes 'that guy is the best thing to ever happen to me and I must get his baby in me ASAP.' She is incapable of doubting her instincts, but she makes up for it by constantly doubting the motives of everyone around her."

The room fell silent as the weight of the words sank in. A painful discussion about how others perceive their mental illness ensued, and while the members of the group drew meaningful connections between similar experiences, the sting of the book lingered. I tried to explain how and why the book was wrong, both in its content and its approach, while also making space for the fact that many medical professionals did in fact think such things. The group members didn't need to be told this, of course; echoes of past interactions with doctors and therapists were quickly brought to mind by the words of the book. It pained me to realize some of those involved my coworkers. It's common in the mental health field to use person-first language such as "a person with schizophrenia" instead of "schizophrenic." We do this to remind our patients and ourselves that no matter the diagnosis, we are all human beings worthy of dignity and respect. This is so commonly observed so as to pass unnoticed, yet team meetings at that job often included mention of difficult "borderlines," usually in reference to those gathered in that very room.

I wrote at length in *This City Is Killing Me* about the lingering stigma associated with the diagnosis of borderline personality disorder through the lens of my client Jacqueline, who was not a member of that group but had many of the same experiences.

It is safe to say that borderline personality disorder is one of the few diagnoses that even seasoned mental health professionals will wince at and hesitate to take on as a client. Nearly every client I see in my private practice with such a diagnosis reveals it to me in hushed tones during our initial phone consultation, bracing for the inevitable rejection.

To be borderline is to occupy a liminal space, unsure of the path forward. Pop songs talk about relationships on the borderline, tilting erratically between the promise of ecstasy and the fear of falling apart. In an age of increasing nationalism, the borderline is a place to be fortified, guarded, to protect the supposed sanctity of the nation-state. Both describe a sort of contested space, neither here nor there. All of us may be able to imagine this sort of state in our relational patterns or countries of residence, but what does it mean to apply such concepts to our minds?

Borderline is a concept dating to the days when psychoanalysis dominated the psychiatric mainstream. For most of his career, Freud was interested in treating neurotics (this before the advent of person-first language, of course), the sort of everyday anxious and depressed people that continue to make up the majority of mental health patients. The other side of the spectrum included the psychotics, those whose perception and way of being in the world was fundamentally different from what the majority experienced. Freud thought psychotics were incapable of being psychoanalyzed, and while other practitioners dating to the first few decades of psychoanalytic thought believed otherwise, all agreed that their treatment looked quite different. Some patients seemed to be in the unstable middle, not entirely psychotic but also with problems beyond pure neurosis. These patients existed in the borderlines between the two categories, hence the name.

Neurotics and psychotics each present with their own difficulties, but they at least can be named, and there is some predictability to the ways they act and how their symptoms manifest. The borderline lacks such stability, a sense of a continuity of character from one moment to the next. In the borderline, one can never know what they are getting into, both for the patient and the mental health professional. The ways in which persons with BPD are talked about in the literature often reinforce this "borderline" status.

While our diagnostic nomenclature has moved beyond the neurotic-psychotic binary, borderline personality disorder continues to share some core features from its days on the psychoanalytic continuum: the need to attach to others as transitional objects, a distorted sense of self and others, fears of abandonment. Along the way toward scientific respectability, it became attached to a series of diagnoses: at first it was placed on the schizophrenia spectrum, later it became linked to depression. It has long been "an adjective in search of a noun," in the words of one famous paper.[1] For the past forty years, it has been a part of a cluster of diagnoses known as personality disorders.

Prior to *DSM-5*, these disorders were kept separate from the other diagnoses grouped along Axis I and placed in their own category, Axis II. While this is no longer the case, personality disorders remain profoundly different from most other mental disorders. Personality disorders shape the way one experiences and interacts with the world; they become attached to one's self in a way we don't normally think of when we talk about depression or schizophrenia. With those disorders, there is a clear before, a sense of self that extends beyond the experience of the illness, and with time and treatment this sense of personhood is hopefully restored (at least to some degree). Clients with personality disorders, though, usually report that they have always been this way. Their symptoms might increase or change somewhat over time, but they usually can't remember a time when their life wasn't impacted by their diagnosis, even before they first heard the name.

None of this means that people with the symptoms of borderline personality disorder are incapable of being treated. Contrary to the assumptions of many, including mental health professionals, the disorder responds well to treatment,[2] often with Dialectical Behavior Therapy or another approach designed to help patients better understand the emotional lives of others. People with the disorder often suffer terribly, so this is undeniably good news. The stigma attached to the diagnosis, though, has yet to catch up.

The most common adjectives used to describe people with borderline personality disorder include manipulative, needy, seductive, and fearful of being rejected and willing to do almost anything to avoid it. Women with characteristics of borderline personality disorder dominated the erotic thrillers that thrived at the box office in the late 1980s and early 1990s. Consider Glenn Close's character, Alex Forrest, in *Fatal Attraction*. After having a fling with Michael Douglas's character, Dan Gallagher, who is married and has a family, she claims that she is pregnant, attempts suicide in front of him, begins stalking him, and kills the family rabbit before attempting to kill Dan's wife. Other fictional portraits are more nuanced, like the main character in the television show *Crazy Ex-Girlfriend*, but with perhaps that exception, people with borderline personality disorder are rarely allowed to be fully human, instead relegated to a barely animated catalog of threatening symptoms that often have to be met with violence to spare their victims from further machinations.

As Susan Sontag argued in her *Illness as Metaphor*, both physical and mental distress are placed within narratives that shape how they are experienced and how we talk about those experiences. Not all diagnoses are seen to subsume one's subjectivity in the manner of a personality disorder. You *experience* depression; you *have* schizophrenia; you *are* borderline. We speak of those who experience most mental illnesses as struggling or suffering from them, but when it comes to the language we use for borderline personality disorder we mostly focus upon its impact upon us: we are the ones allegedly being manipulated, seduced, clung to. No other mental disorder is so focused upon the impact the person with the diagnosis has upon others.

Our focus on the impact people with borderline personality disorder have upon us elides an important fact: we all manipulate and cling to others. By writing these words on a page, I am hoping to offer something compelling to my readers to gain their attention. I have those in my life whom I cannot imagine living without. The implicit critique in assigning these qualities to people with borderline personality disorder is that they aren't that good at them. I recall a client from my former DBT group who often got into disputes with other group members, usually due to her becoming too reliant upon them outside of our sessions. In pain and desperation she would reach out, they would inevitably fail her in some way, and she would respond with fury, papering over a deeper sense of hurt. Every time this happened, and it happened often, she would try to steer the subject discussed that week back toward a barely veiled critique of the person whom she believed had wronged her. This was all quite transparent; she and many others with BPD had not learned the subtler ways in which we try to influence others.

I cannot deny that she and other people with borderline personality disorder suffer—I have seen it too often to believe otherwise—yet the ways in which we conceive of the diagnosis shape our experience of it beyond what the concept of stigma can capture. There is something else vitally important to consider when it comes to the concept of borderline personality disorder: gender. As late as the *DSM-IV-TR* (2000), it was thought that three times as many women merit the diagnosis as do men. While it is now assumed that men and women experience the disorder in equal proportion, the majority of patients seeking treatment for the disorder continue to be women. Men with the diagnosis present differently, tending to have an explosive temperament, engage in frequent risk-taking, and have substance use problems.[3] These are serious issues, to be sure, but for most people, even mental health professionals, this doesn't sound like what we are trained to recognize as borderline personality disorder. Many of these men most likely end up with a diagnosis of bipolar disorder, itself a subject of stigma but not nearly to the same degree. The prototypical borderline patient is almost always coded as feminine.

Consider again the symptoms of borderline personality disorder. An unstable sense of self, fears of abandonment, difficulties maintaining relationships, self-harm behaviors, mood instability, feeling empty, dissociation, outbursts of anger, impulsivity: if you remove the concept of mental disorder, does this not sound like every patriarchal stereotype of women that you have ever heard? If they are women we don't like, they are crazy, manipulative "bitches"; if these traits are portrayed in a positive light, they are manic pixie dream girls, a term first coined by the film critic Nathan Rabin.

Borderline personality disorder is the most egregious example of a gendered personality disorder, but most of them demonstrate some degree of gender bias. As our understanding of the construction of gender has increased, it has become further evident that traits stereotypically associated with femininity are far more likely to be categorized as a disorder. One study found that male-identified people with a high degree of nonmasculine behavior were more likely to have features of all personality disorders save antisocial when ranked by both themselves and their peers.[4] The same did not hold true for women-identified people with a high degree of nonfeminine behavior, who were seen as having fewer features of a personality disorder by their peers. The implication is clear: no matter one's gender identity, the higher one evinces traits stereotypically associated with femininity, the greater one's chances of ending up with a personality disorder.

If an entire class of disorders appears to have such a strong bias against traits and features typically coded as feminine, it would seem to be ripe for deconstruction. This has been a battle within psychiatry since the early days of psychoanalysis. Do our labels actually say something meaningful about the person in front of us, or do they serve to describe deviations from the norm of the dominant class in order to weed out those in need of correcting? We've already seen how this can work with race. When it comes to considerations of gender, borderline personality disorder is not the first time such labels have been found to have a profound bias. The first great disorder of psychoanalysis, hysteria, functioned in much the same way within the discourse of its time.

Hysteria flourished during the late nineteenth century, but its historical roots stretch back far earlier. The term itself means "wandering womb," and in the classical era of medicine, the womb was thought to be the source of multiple forms of affliction when it became unruly or unregulated. Because it was due to the womb, this of course meant it could only afflict women. Plato writes of this in the *Timaeus*: "whenever the matrix or womb, as it is called,—which is an indwelling creature desirous of child-bearing,—remains without fruit long beyond the due season, it is vexed and takes it ill; and by straying all ways through the body and blocking up the passages of the breath and preventing respiration it casts the body into the uttermost distress, and causes, moreover, all kinds of maladies."

During the medieval era, the sort of symptoms later associated with hysteria were less associated with a renegade uterus and instead were thought to be signs of demonic possession or affliction. The first "victims" of the witchcraft epidemic that plagued Salem, Massachusetts, in 1692, Elizabeth Parris and Abigail Williams, began screaming, throwing objects, uttering strange sounds, and contorting themselves into strange positions. Had they been born a few centuries later, they would have been thought to be hysterical, but within the discourse of their era, they were under assault by the devil himself. Because they were the victims in this construction, "treatment" focused on punishing those responsible for causing such symptoms.

When people in the seventeenth century were not attributing illnesses to supernatural evil, they began to turn to the nervous system rather than the uterus. Hysteria joined other nascent mental illnesses such as mania, melancholia, and lunacy as a disorder of the nerves. Just as we saw with neurasthenia earlier, it took a certain sort of social class and degree of mental activity to have one's nerves impacted. As physician George Cheyne wrote in his *The English Malady* (1733), "Fools, weak or stupid Persons, heavy and dull Souls, are seldom troubled with Vapours or Lowness of Spirits." While hysteria was still seen as a predominantly feminine affliction, it became something that could afflict men as well. It also morphed from a pernicious affliction to something that impacted the overworked working class, anticipating the first diagnosis of neurasthenia almost a century later.

By the time that came about, the discourse began to shift, and hysteria was again seen as a feminine malady at the same time that its social status underwent a profound evolution. The same rhetoric used in our era to describe people with borderline personality disorder was used at the time to describe women with hysteria: they demanded too much attention from their doctors, were often resistant to treatment, had an exhibitionist streak, and had be confronted in a stern manner in order to be shaken out of their stupor. The medical establishment of the Victorian era was already hostile to women; hysteria gave them one more tool to medicalize women's suffering so that it would not have to be taken seriously and instead serve as further evidence of their status as the "weaker" sex. Some treatments largely relegated to the fringes of medicine proposed confronting this supposed imbalance head-on, removing the clitoris or the ovaries. While radical, these alleged "cures" merely took the present-day understanding of hysteria to its logical end—curing the woman by removing all evidence of her womanhood.

Jean-Martin Charcot, a nineteenth-century French neurologist, proposed a different method. Charcot ruled over the Salpêtrière in Paris, a public hospital filled with poor women who could not receive care elsewhere, for over thirty years. Before Charcot turned to hysteria, he played a key role in identifying multiple sclerosis and amyotrophic lateral sclerosis (ALS, known for a time as Charcot's disease in France), establishing his medical bona fides. Charcot was insistent that hysteria was neurological in origin and was particularly suited to a form of cure that relaxed one's nervous system and suspended some of one's critical faculties: hypnosis.

Charcot made regular presentations of his patients that anyone could attend, and as his fame grew, these became society affairs not just in France but across the whole of Europe. Charcot would use hypnosis to demonstrate how the power of suggestion could bend the wills of his hysterical patients, both as a method of cure and also to demonstrate his power over them. Charcot was also interested in the then-new art of photography, and under his watch, pictures of his patients in the throes of their illness, often in semi-erotic poses, were widely disseminated. While Charcot believed that hysteria did not discriminate amongst genders, his work on male hysteria attracted far less interest or notice.

In 1885, a young Austrian neurologist traveled to Paris for a three-month fellowship with Charcot. Inspired to continue his own study of hysteria based on Charcot's method, Sigmund Freud entered private practice the following year and began to experiment with hypnosis. While he would later abandon the method, he remained fascinated with the diagnosis and devoted the earliest part of his psychoanalytic career to finding a cure. His first major published work, coauthored with an older physician and mentor named Josef Breuer, was *Studies on Hysteria* (1895). In this work and elsewhere, Freud would claim that the suffering of the person with hysteria was psychological rather than physical in origin. Long gone are any notions of errant uteruses or demonic possession, cementing the turn toward our own psychiatric era.

The case that drew the most attention out of the five included in the book was that of Anna O., a woman Breuer had treated periodically from 1880 to 1882. Anna O., real name Bertha Pappenheim, began experiencing a variety of remarkable symptoms including hallucinations, aphasia, paralysis, mood swings, being unable to speak anything other than English (her native language being German), and disordered eating, beginning when her father fell ill and worsening after his death. Breuer utilized hypnosis and found that in this altered state, Pappenheim felt free to talk about her experiences and seemed to have more access to deeper motivations for her behavior. Pappenheim called this process "chimney sweeping" or "the talking cure." Breuer abandoned Charcot's use of hypnotic suggestion, instead using Pappenheim's lowered defenses to enlist her as a co-laborer in her cure.

In one representative passage, Breuer notes that during the peak of summer, Pappenheim suddenly found herself unable to drink water, subsisting on fruits but remaining constantly parched. She could not isolate the cause of this hydrophobia until, under hypnosis, "she grumbled about her English lady-companion whom she did not care for, and went on to describe, with every sign of disgust, how she had once gone into that lady's room and how her little dog—horrid creature!—had drunk out of a glass there. The patient had said nothing, as she had wanted to be polite. After giving further energetic expression to the anger she had held back, she asked for something to drink, drank a large quantity of water without any difficulty and woke from her hypnosis with the glass at her lips; and thereupon the disturbance vanished, never to return." This became a pattern; under hypnosis, Pappenheim would uncover the trigger for her symptoms, and, having been told by Breuer what she had said upon rising out of the hypnotic state, found her symptoms abated. Breuer continued in such a manner until he declared the case closed. It should also be noted that, in real life, Pappenheim did not achieve such a tidy resolution to her suffering as Breuer claimed. She was referred by him to a sanatorium a week after he declared her cured. She would later find peace and became a pioneering social worker in her home country of Germany.

In *Studies on Hysteria*, Freud theorized there was a part of our memories that actively worked to keep painful events from surfacing. Hypnosis allowed some access to them, but free association worked even better, he came to believe, because it enlisted the patient more directly in their recovery. The problem of hysteria was that the person suffered from their own memories, to paraphrase the early Freud's formulation. In this regard, Freud drew quite close to the modern understanding of trauma, but this was not to last. Within the span of a few years, he grew less comfortable with the idea that hysterical suffering was rooted in sexual trauma, substituting instead a maelstrom of conflicting psychosexual impulses. We can see this new perspective at work in Freud's treatment of Dora (Ida Bauer), a young woman of eighteen whom Freud saw in 1900 for occasional loss of voice, persistent cough, and social isolation.

Freud first met with Dora's father, who informed Freud of the history of Dora's symptoms and provided some background information. Dora's father noted that his family was particularly close to another couple, Herr and Frau K. Dora enjoyed spending time with them and their children until she reported to her father that Herr K had made an indecent "proposal" to her. Her father confronted Herr K, who denied doing anything untoward. Freud notes his evolution from the earlier position that hysteria was rooted in real traumatic incidents, for "there is the further consideration that some of these symptoms (the cough and the loss of voice) had been produced by the patient years before the time of the trauma, and that their earliest appearances belong to her childhood, since they occurred in her eighth year. If, therefore, the trauma theory is not to be abandoned, we must go back to her childhood and look about there for any influences or impressions which might have had an effect *analogous to that of a trauma*" (emphasis mine). The search becomes less about events as they actually happened and instead about what effect they had upon Dora due to her interpretation of them.

When Freud spoke with Dora, he heard a very different story. Dora revealed that her father had been having an affair with Frau K, and she felt that he had pawned her off on Herr K as some perverse form of recompense. Dora later related another incident with Herr K to Freud, telling him that when she was fourteen, he cornered her and kissed her without her consent. Freud is less interested in what to us is an obvious violation than in Dora's reaction to it, for he sees in her disgust a sign that hysterical symptoms were already present: "the behaviour of this child of fourteen was already entirely and completely hysterical. I should without question consider a person hysterical in whom an occasion for sexual excitement elicited feelings that were preponderantly or exclusively unpleasurable; and I should do so whether or no the person were capable of producing somatic symptoms." Freud continued to doggedly insist that the heart of the matter was Dora's attraction to Herr K, her resistance to her feelings, and her jealousy over her father's attachment to Frau K. Eleven weeks into the treatment, Dora broke it off.

Freud deemed her treatment a failure, but not for the reasons you might expect. He believed that, at that time, he was not sufficiently attuned to the dynamics of transference, the ways in which a patient comes to treat their therapist along the same lines as other significant people in their life, and he thus missed this important undercurrent to their work. Soon after he published his case study, Freud's interests began to shift toward neurosis, and for the rest of his lifetime he would largely disregard the condition that so occupied his earlier years.

The next great outbreak of hysteria occurred not in the parlors of European metropolises but in the trenches of World War I. Many of the same symptoms once deemed hysterical began to appear in combat veterans. While they too were first thought to be caused by physical trauma, doctors soon found that their suffering was psychological in origin. The entire edifice of hysteria began to slowly melt away and became a historical curiosity.

The twin world wars accelerated this shift. The violence caused many of the founding figures of psychoanalysis to flee to England and the United States, since Freud and several of his colleagues were Jewish and directly threatened by Nazi violence. The impact of so much violence also greatly increased the roll of potential patients. Most practitioners began to focus their work away from the sort of long-term institutionalized treatment that hysteria often required to outpatient clinics, just as we earlier saw with schizophrenia.

So what happened to all of those with hysteria? Did they become borderline cases overnight? Diagnostic transitions are rarely so neat. There are probably some patients seen today whose symptoms would be considered hysteria had they been treated a century ago. Others never make it to a psychiatrist's office and instead go to their primary care doctor and, if they are not dismissed outright, receive a diagnosis such as chronic fatigue syndrome. Whether the symptoms are located in the mind or located in the body, though, the overwhelming reaction on the part of the medical community is skepticism and blame.[5]

The author Lauren Hillenbrand describes her medical journey with chronic fatigue syndrome in terms not dissimilar to those of hysteria. At age nineteen, she suddenly lost all her energy, along with a great deal of weight, and also experienced fevers, chills, exhaustion, swollen lymph nodes, and dizziness. Unsure what to do, she went to see her old pediatrician, who told her she had strep and referred her to an internist. The internist referred her to a psychiatrist, but when that psychiatrist told her that her condition was physical and not mental, the internist told her to find another psychiatrist. This second psychiatrist suggested that what she was experiencing was a revolt against growing up: "Laura, everyone goes through this. . . . It's a normal adjustment to adulthood. You'll grow out of it in a few years." Hillenbrand later requested her notes to find he had written "Couldn't handle school. Dropped out." Several months later, she would finally receive a diagnosis of chronic fatigue syndrome, shedding relationships, future prospects, and almost all of her hope for the future along the way.[6]

People find a way of speaking even when their words are dismissed. Sometimes this takes the form of desperate actions to avoid feeling abandoned while contending with an inner sense of desperate aloneness; at other times it is a young woman ceasing to speak because when she tells her father about her sexual assault, he believes her abuser instead of her. Borderline personality disorder and hysteria are both often found at the margins, sometimes literally in the case of Charcot's patients but also among women in a patriarchal age who, despite their privilege, are treated as little more than accessories to the ambitions of the men who surround them. For many like Dora, it proved more advantageous to fall silent rather than continue to fight to have one's experiences validated and, hopefully, treated.

A psychiatric diagnosis too often shapes how we listen to the person sitting in front of us. Once they are revealed to have hysteria or borderline personality disorder, everything that they might have to say only functions as confirmation of their diagnosis. So many of the patients in that DBT group had horror stories of how they had been treated by mental health professionals once they disclosed their diagnosis. This damages not just those suffering mentally but also those like Hillenbrand who have no significant psychiatric symptoms but are assumed to be mentally ill in some way because that seems to be the easiest explanation for what they're reporting. I have seen more than a few cases like Hillenbrand in my years of practice, both men and women presenting with a constellation of admittedly confusing symptoms that one of their doctors has become convinced only resides in their head.

Thus far, we have seen how notions of class, race, and gender have shaped psychiatric discourse from the beginning.

Now we will turn to perhaps the most famous discarded diagnosis—the ones whose main purpose was to police the boundaries of sexuality.

CHAPTER 4
"THEY CALL US QUEER, YOU CALL US SICK"

When the COVID-19 pandemic forced my practice online, I was surprised by some of the unexpected ways in which my work shifted. At a fundamental level, therapy is two people talking together, and while stuttering internet connections and random background noise could sometimes make that difficult, I found my clients to be generous in their patience and we were able to make it work. Such minor inconveniences were certainly better than risking infection, of course, and the elaborate precautions my clients and I would have to take to meet in person seemed far more onerous. What I found that I was missing, though, was everything else that surrounded those conversations. Our bodies communicate volumes before we speak, and now that I couldn't easily observe the slump in someone's shoulders, the cast to their eyes, the way that they transitioned from my waiting room to my office, I found myself trying to gather such information in other ways.

Harper was one such client, someone I used to see in person and then quickly transitioned to virtual once the pandemic took hold. Harper was a master's student in public policy in the final year of the program, and when I first met Harper, they presented as a cisgender male. One of Harper's favorite pursuits outside of academia was bodybuilding, and they would often come to our appointments straight from the gym. Our initial work together centered upon their anxiety, a struggle that the pandemic would soon kick into high gear. Harper had seen a few women since we started working together, both one-night stands and longer relationships, and they were currently seeing a fellow student. The pandemic seemed to accelerate their relationship; in order to continue seeing each other, they moved in together a few months after they began dating.

We were discussing the course of their relationship one session when Harper off-handedly mentioned to me, "My girlfriend and I were taking a walk the other day and we passed this guy. She turned to me and said, 'I think he's kinda hot.' I told her that I thought so too, and she seemed only sort of surprised." That was how Harper came out to me as queer.

When it comes to such disclosures with friends or family members, many choose to come out directly through a conversation. In my own work, though, I've found statements like Harper's to be far more common; brief shots across the bow that test my reaction and see if I'm someone that's safe. It's vitally important to be aware of such moments, for while they might seem like passing comments to me, they are often the product of no small degree of internal wrangling, and the vulnerability inherent in such discussions means that my immediate reaction will crystallize for them whether or not I am someone they can talk to about such things. If they find that I am not, the therapeutic relationship will likely be irreparably shattered.

That statement marked a shift in my own perception of Harper from a muscle-bound paragon of masculinity to something else entirely. It was a few sessions later when Harper casually brushed some hair back from their face that I noticed they had painted their nails. I made a remark about liking the color, and that led us to a wider conversation about their gender identity. Over several sessions, we explored their questions about it, the ways in which they had attempted to evade such questions over the years. Harper was intensely bright, so my function was more as a guide than anything else. After some time weighing the various options open to them in terms of identity and expression, they settled upon a nongendered form of their birth name and they/them pronouns.

Being transgender is never easy, and as a cisgender man, I cannot fathom the myriad of ways in which our transphobic society makes life difficult for those who fail to conform to our rigid gender expectations. That being said, I was quite impressed by how calm and happy Harper felt. They already had trans friends, so the idea was not new to them, and while their journey was by no means easy, they felt surrounded by loving and supportive friends and family. When I compared their story to an earlier client of mine, Jacqueline (whom I wrote about extensively in *This City Is Killing Me*), the differences in their experience were remarkable. Jacqueline came out decades earlier in a family that was at first strongly resistant and only barely supportive now, and their refusal to accept her had profound consequences for her life and her mental health. In neither of their cases did I feel that their gender identity was itself a product of their thought patterns or mental illness, but in that instance, the *DSM* would disagree with me.

If a person has a strong desire to be a gender other than the one they were assigned at birth, feels an incongruence between their assigned gender and their sense of self, has a strong desire for the characteristics of another gender, and feels that one responds to situations and others in a manner fitting a gender other than the one they are assigned, they may qualify for a diagnosis known as gender dysphoria. There is one other significant symptom that must be present, however: the above symptoms must cause them clinically significant distress. The idea here, then, is that a child who was assigned female at birth but has felt they were a male as long as they can remember, has taken steps to present and react like a male, and feels no distress about any of that would not qualify. Someone like Harper, then, would not fulfill this requirement, but someone like Jacqueline would.

The first and second editions of the *DSM* included no diagnosis addressing this category of experience. It first appeared in the third edition (1980) where it was labeled "gender identity disorder" under the general category of psychosexual disorders and was only used for children. Adults with similar concerns were diagnosed with "transsexualism." In a revision of the third edition (1987), an additional category called "gender identity disorder of adolescence and adulthood, non-transsexual type" was added. The category was made a little cleaner in the fourth edition (1994), reducing the available options to gender identity disorder in adolescents and adults or gender identity disorder in children. In the most recent fifth edition, the name was changed to gender dysphoria in an effort to avoid the pejorative connotations of the word "disorder."

Despite eliminating the word "disorder" from the diagnosis, it remains inescapable that the criteria for gender dysphoria are in a book called the *Diagnostic and Statistical Manual of Mental*

Disorders; no amount of rhetorical softening can alter this fact. One could argue that the diagnosis is there to help those who feel distress at their perceived gender incongruence, not those who are content to identify as transgender. This relies upon the assumption, though, that home environments and societies are relatively stable across patients. The *DSM* knows this is not true, of course, noting, "Distress may not be manifest in social environments supportive of the child's desire to live in the role of the other gender and may emerge only if the desire is interfered with . . . distress may, however, be mitigated by supportive environments and knowledge that biomedical treatments exist to reduce incongruence." Acknowledging this does not change the fact that a transgender individual from a hostile household could easily land the diagnosis while a person from a more progressive one could not, with the only significant difference being their social surround.

There is another option for the clinician treating a transgender patient. In the current *DSM*, gender dysphoria is assigned its own category, an island unto its own. Flip forward a few hundred pages, however, and you will land upon the paraphilic disorders. Paraphilias, in general, are disorders where someone receives sexual excitement and/or stimulation from something generally not seen as erotic. This includes the criminal (voyeurism, exhibitionism, frotteurism, pedophilia), kinks (bondage, sadomasochism, fetishes), and, at the end of the section, a diagnosis named transvestic disorder. Transvestic disorder can be diagnosed if an individual experiences recurrent and intense sexual arousal from cross-dressing over a period of six months and experiences distress or impairment as a result of it. The disorder can be further modified "with fetishism" if the person is sexually aroused by the materials of the garments themselves or "with autogynephilia" if the person is aroused by imagining themselves as female.

It doesn't take much imagination to see how this could be weaponized in the hands of a nonaffirming medical professional. It allows trans people to be labeled as mentally ill if they dress in clothes not corresponding to their natal gender as long as they meet the criteria of being disturbed by this fact and are sexually aroused in some way by it. Again, clinically significant distress is far from a benign concept, and it isn't hard to see how a hostile clinician could attribute arousal to a trans person exploring their identity. Indeed, the concept aligns with the general societal stigma of trans individuals as being sex-obsessed, whether it's the specter of the trans woman "invading" women's bathrooms for the purposes of sexual assault or the cisgender fascination with the genitals of trans people. If I thought that Harper's gender exploration was not healthy because of my own biases and misconceptions, and if they continued to tell me how they felt their exploration of femininity felt erotic, I would have more than enough ammunition to diagnose them with a serious mental illness.

I want to take a step back from the particular diagnosis of transvestic disorder to consider the class of paraphilas in general. When considered together, it is not immediately clear what they all have in common that lands them in their shared category. Some are now broadly recognized as expressions of sexuality that, with proper consent, can be exercised between willing participants (BDSM). Others may not be as broadly accepted but are generally seen as harmless (all manners of fetishes), while the remainder cannot be expressed without both committing a crime and violating society's standards for healthy sexual expression (exhibitionism, pedophilia). How does this disparate group somehow cohere into a discrete category? They only make sense if you view them as clustered around an absence, negations of an unspoken standard.

That standard is procreative sex. All the paraphilias are defined by sexual excitement by something other than sex aimed at procreation, and many of them have been associated with the LGBTQ community in the past. The inclusion of BDSM does not rule out straight people, but it is notable that expressions of sexuality that have not been coded as queer (e.g., masturbation) have long been normalized within psychiatric discourse. The logic of the paraphilias continues to exercise a powerful normative function over sex, defining that which is normal and that which is disordered. It is the same logic, coincidentally, that landed homosexuality in the *DSM*.

The idea of male homosexuality represented a test case for many of the earliest thinkers at the beginning of the age of psychology. In Richard von Krafft-Ebing's highly influential *Psychopathia Sexualis* (1886), he contended that homosexuality was a sign of degeneracy, reflecting his Darwinian viewpoint that nonprocreative sex in general was pathological.[1] Each case study he included traced the development of a "perverse" sexual instinct to earlier faults in the family tree, mental illness and substance abuse among them but also including such conditions as epilepsy and other physical disorders. This echoes the logic of the paraphilias, but none other than Sigmund Freud challenged this view. Freud noted that gay desire seemed equally distributed across all social classes so it in itself was not sufficient to cause degeneracy.

Freud wavered theoretically in his beliefs about gay people and their psychology, but his general stance was as follows: all of us began life as bisexual and through our experiences tended toward either the opposite or the same sex when it comes to attraction. Freud did believe that gay desire represented a deviation from the course of normal development, but that in itself was not a cause for alarm. He disdained the idea of what we would now call conversion therapy, believing at most it could enable a gay person to feel attraction toward the opposite sex (due to all of us starting out as bisexual) but could never eliminate their biologically determined queerness. Freud's practice reflected this relative openness. He resisted the efforts of his followers to bar gay analysts from psychoanalytic groups, not exactly offering a full-throated endorsement of them but denying that being gay must always be an impediment to analytic practice. In a now-famous 1935 letter to an American woman who wrote him asking what to do with her gay son, he replied: "Homosexuality is assuredly no advantage, but it is nothing to be ashamed of, no vice, no degradation; it cannot be classified as an illness; we consider it to be a variation of the sexual function, produced by a certain arrest of sexual development. Many highly respectable individuals of ancient and modern times have been homosexuals, several of the greatest men among them. (Plato, Michelangelo, Leonardo da Vinci, etc). It is a great injustice to persecute homosexuality as a crime—and a cruelty, too." It may have helped that his daughter Anna, who would go on to become an influential psychoanalyst in her own right, was a lesbian, a fact he probably knew as he analyzed her twice (an obvious violation of ethical norms, both then and now).

After Freud's death, psychoanalysis lost its figurehead, and those who followed questioned some of the central tenets of his system. Sandor Rado, a Hungarian psychoanalyst who practiced in America for the majority of his career, challenged

Freud's notion of essential bisexuality.[2] Rado was a gender essentialist and believed that the male-female pairing was the only "natural" option, writing, "the sexes are an outcome of evolutionary differentiation of contrasting yet complementary reproductive systems. Aside from the so-called hermaphrodite . . . every individual is either male or female. The view that each individual is both male and female (either more male or less female or the other way around) . . . has no scientific foundation."[3] If we were not born bisexual, being queer was not a fork in the developmental road but rather a profound deviation from the natural order of things. Because everyone was thus incipiently straight, therapy need not be so pessimistic regarding the possibility of changing one's sexual desire, giving birth to the possibility of conversion therapy.

Rado provided the theory, and another analyst named Irving Bieber sought to provide the data. A 1962 study headed by Bieber, titled *Homosexuality* and published under the auspices of the New York Society of Medical Psychoanalysts, compared 106 homosexual patients to 100 heterosexual patients in an effort to illuminate where the former's development went wrong. Bieber reported that gay men had a close, restrictive relationship with their mother at roughly two times the rate as that of straight men, and their relationships with their fathers were often detached and hostile. These conditions, Bieber believed, combined to create the gay male. Other researchers, notably Alfred Kinsey, disagreed on both theoretical and empirical grounds, but Bieber's work proved to be dominant at the time.

Rado, Bieber, and other prominent voices in the homosexuality-as-disorder camp believed that the primary problem afflicting the gay person was a phobia of heterosexuality, and their treatment was thus oriented toward confronting and resolving these fears. They viewed this as an act of compassion, believing that true satisfaction in a gay relationship was an illusory goal destined to frustrate and disappoint. It also seems of note that the specter of the gay male loomed particularly large in their formulations; lesbians did not seem to rate nearly the same level of concern. Thus, homosexuality came to be included in the *DSM*, first classified as a sociopathic personality disturbance in the first edition (1952) and reclassified as a sexual deviation in the subsequent one (1968), numbered amongst the paraphilias.

The second edition of the *DSM* was released into a profoundly different world than the first. The Stonewall Uprising, which took place the year after publication, is often seen as the beginning of the modern gay rights movement. Protests against the dominant psychiatric position on homosexuality had been ongoing but sporadic until the movement became both more radicalized and more united, shifting from a focus upon individual practitioners and their research to the overarching idea of homosexuality as a mental illness. When the American Psychiatric Association decided to hold their annual conference in San Francisco in 1970, a group of gay activists began to formulate a plan to bring the struggle directly to the psychiatrists engaged in their repression.

Some closeted and sympathetic members of the APA passed along press passes to a group of gay people involved in the movement. Bieber was a particular target due to his study, and he was located at a panel discussion on transsexuals and homosexuality. According to an oral history from the activist Gary Alinder, he confronted Bieber.

"You are the pigs who make it possible for the cops to beat homosexuals," Alinder told Bieber. "They call us queer, you—so politely—call us sick."

Alinder says that Bieber responded, "I never said homosexuals were sick, what I said was that they have displaced sexual adjustment."

"That's the same thing, motherfucker," one of Alinder's fellow activists countered.

Bieber replied, "I don't want to oppress homosexuals, I want to liberate them, to liberate them from that which is paining them—their homosexuality."

Alinder ends his account by noting, "That used to be called genocide."[4]

Bieber was reportedly shaken up by this confrontation, which seemed far different than the sort of calm and steady debate about the lives of gay people (amongst straight people, of course) with which he was familiar. Bieber was representative of a type of psychiatrist who believed the work required a certain seriousness coupled with an isolation from the cares of the day. As the turbulent events of the 1960s began to pile up, this detachment began to be seen as a liability amongst several younger psychiatrists who wanted the organization, along with the profession as a whole, to take a more active stance toward the present. These psychiatrists began to meet together regularly to develop a plan for pushing out the old guard of the APA hierarchy by running for office themselves.

Gay rights groups continued to apply pressure from the outside, again storming into the 1971 APA convention in protest. One year later, after some prodding from an activist named Barbara Gittings, the psychiatrist John Fryer appeared on stage at the 1972 convention as Dr. Anonymous. Taking pains to avoid being outed, Fryer was wearing a wig, a Nixon mask, and an oversized tuxedo and had his voice distorted as he talked about his experiences as a gay psychiatrist. He spoke about how the pathologization of homosexuality had hurt him both personally and professionally.

Despite the efforts of Fryer and others, reform might not have happened when it did if not for a chance encounter between activist Ronald Gold and psychiatrist Robert Spitzer, a member of the APA's Committee on Nomenclature that determined what did and did not constitute a mental illness. After Gold and others interrupted a 1972 behavioral therapy convention Spitzer was attending, Spitzer was annoyed but intrigued and agreed to help Gold set up a meeting with his committee. Spitzer also organized a 1973 debate between gay activists and the homosexuality-as-disorder camp at that year's convention. As Gold later told *This American Life,* he believed that it was not due to either of those two events that homosexuality was removed from the *DSM* but instead attributed it to an evening at a tiki bar following the debate.

Gold was allied with a shadow group of gay psychiatrists, the "GAYPA," who held an annual party following the convention. Since being gay could cost any of them their livelihoods, the gathering was a clandestine affair. Gold decided to invite Spitzer along so he could gain perspective on the issue aside from theoretical debates. Spitzer's presence was not exactly welcome, but his invite had the intended effect when an Army psychiatrist joined the group after hearing Gold speak earlier in the day, bursting into tears when he realized that he was not alone. According to Gold, Spitzer returned to his hotel room that evening and wrote the resolution to remove homosexuality from the *DSM.*[5]

Spitzer did not entirely strike homosexuality from the *DSM* in 1973; rather, he created a new category for those who experienced distress due to their perceived sexual orientation. In the revised second edition, this diagnosis was known as "sexual orientation disturbance" and later rechristened "ego dystonic homosexuality" in the third edition until all trace of it was removed in 1987. Until then, one could still be diagnosed as mentally ill solely for the fact of being gay, and all manner of conversion therapies meant to address this "pathology" were thereby legitimated.

The same logic currently at work in the diagnosis of gender dysphoria is that which supported the idea of an ego dystonic sexual orientation, psychoanalytic speak for a part of one's personality not in accord with how one wishes to be perceived. The experience of a gay person can differ wildly depending upon where they live, but most of us would now attribute this disparity to the degree of homophobia present in a given area rather than anything internal to the individual. We have not yet made it this far, though, when the person is trans.

The battle over homosexuality and the *DSM* is not ancient history. Psychiatry is one of the oldest specialties in medicine; over half of practicing psychiatrists are over the age of fifty-five.[6] While most psychiatrists today probably weren't practicing at the time of the debate, they were trained by those who were. It comes as no surprise then that the stance of the psychiatric mainstream toward less prominent expressions of gender and sexuality continues to be relatively conservative.

It is absolutely appropriate that the APA only reversed course when it came into contact with gay people who gave no evidence of being distressed or disordered by their sexuality, but this had the unfortunate side effect of leaving the logical structure of the paraphilias intact. Psychiatry made no sustained effort to confront the style of reasoning that led them to become the self-appointed arbiter of normative sexuality, so the exact same thought process remains intact. When examined more closely, however, the same gaps and fissures are at work.

The section of *DSM-5* addressing sexual and gender identity disorders was chaired by Kenneth Zucker. The National Gay and Lesbian Task Force expressed concern about Zucker's appointment to chair of the work group, as well as that of another member, Ray Blanchard, for what they characterized as their outdated, even harmful, views on gender. Blanchard's contribution to the concept of gender dysphoria is autogynephilia, the previously mentioned modifier for the diagnosis of transvestic disorder that was included as a feature of gender identity disorder in *DSM-IV-TR*. Blanchard developed a taxonomy in 1989 that separated trans women into two distinct groups. Androphilic trans women, whom he thought were actually feminine gay men who transitioned to attract straight men, were supposedly separate from gynephilic, bisexual, and asexual trans women, whose attraction to women competes with an attraction to oneself as a woman.[7]

By the time Blanchard was appointed to the working group, this thesis had been severely challenged empirically, but aside from having no basis in reality, it seemingly confirms lingering stereotypes about trans women. Blanchard has a fairly active Twitter presence, and many of his tweets seem to confirm the suspicion that his theory is rooted in transphobia. On August 10, 2020, he tweeted, "Pronouns used to tell you a person's sex. Now they tell you a person's politics." A few days earlier, he tweeted out a link for self-identified autogynephiles to connect on 4chan. I didn't have to dig back into his feed to find these; they happened to be the two most recent tweets when I began writing this chapter.

It's not exactly hard to see what Blanchard is up to, but his was not even the most controversial assignment. That designation belongs to its aforementioned chair Kenneth Zucker. For many years, Zucker was the psychologist-in-chief at Toronto's Center for Addiction and Mental Health and headed up its Gender Identity Clinic. Zucker has a particular approach to the treatment of transgender children that is highly controversial. In an NPR article summarizing his approach, Zucker instructs the parents of a child assigned male at birth with a pronounced interest in feminine characteristics to banish all "girlish" toys and prevent him from playing with girls. For children under ten, Zucker's approach is to make the child more comfortable with the gender they were assigned at birth based upon his belief that gender identity remains fluid until roughly that age. When pressed about the comparison between being transgender and being gay, which would make his approach akin to conversion therapy, Zucker rejected the analogy, saying, "Suppose you were a clinician and a four-year-old Black kid came into your office and said he wanted to be white. Would you go with that? . . . I don't think we would."[8] For Zucker, being transgender can cause a lifetime of difficulties, and the proper clinical approach is to help steer children away from this harsh reality if at all possible.

While Zucker's approach was once acceptable practice for treating transgender children, the tides have shifted in recent years to emphasize children's agency in shaping their gender expression. Critics accused Zucker of practicing conversion therapy under a different name, and in February 2015, the

Center for Addiction and Mental Health commissioned an external review of the Gender Identity Clinic's practices. Ten months later, they presented Zucker with the review's findings, promptly firing him and winding down the clinic's operations.

Zucker's firing triggered a flurry of articles on all sides of the debate. Trans activists and allies hailed the move as another step on the way toward dismantling transphobia in medicine, while others contended that the hospital had given into political pressure and silenced the vital and important work that Zucker was doing alongside his colleagues. One of Zucker's most ardent defenders was Jesse Singal, a cisgender journalist who has written on transgender issues for years, often with a pronounced skeptical tinge.

Singal makes his perspective clear in the opening paragraphs of his February 7, 2016, article for *The Cut* titled "How the Fight Over Transgender Kids Got a Leading Sex Researcher Fired":[9] "[I]f you look closely at what really happened . . . it's hard not to come to an uncomfortable, politically incorrect conclusion: Zucker's defenders are right. This was a show trial." Singal refers to a statistic about desistance rates amongst children with dysphoria that found almost 75 percent of them eventually return to the gender they were assigned at birth. This would indeed be shocking if true, but that statistic includes those in the study who did not return to the clinic. There is no good reason to take this as sufficient evidence that they desisted, and Singal later noted the error, tweeting "I done goofed."[10] Singal also cited an anonymous clinician from the GIC who expressed concern that trans children who want to desist might be pressured into remaining trans if their parents get involved in advocacy work, if they come out to their school and classmates, and so forth. As a parent, this strikes me as deeply confusing. Our basement is littered with the toys and hobbies of ages past, and while that can indeed be annoying, at no point did I consider forcing my daughter to play more with her expensive handmade doll or ride her scooter. To be a child or adolescent is to be in perpetual flux, picking up hobbies, interests, and identities to find out what feels right, what feels like home. This can happen with sports, with music, and yes, with gender and sexuality, but at no point does any good parent insist that their child keep their hair blue or stay on the soccer team long after their interest has withered.

The external review of the GIC's practices was later challenged for making some false claims about Zucker's practice, and Singal is able to unearth evidence to support these claims. It is not necessary for Zucker to be a traumatizing monster, however, for his practices and those of his clinic to be harmful. At root, Zucker's approach believes that this is a hard world for trans children, and they would be better able to thrive in every way if they were cisgender. Perhaps this held some truth when his work began, but that is no longer the case now. The same logic, incidentally, has been used in conversion therapies of all sorts, whether it is for gender or for sexuality. Attempting to shape a child's gender expression toward a more normative form stifles the growing voices of children and communicates to them that they are able to explore only so far, that only certain ways of being in the world are okay. That strikes me as an exceedingly dangerous message to communicate to a developing mind, far more insidious than letting them play with nail polish or dolls in the process of becoming who they are.

Singal's article is notable for what it doesn't include: the voices of trans children or of parents who found fault with

Zucker's approach. The trans writers Parker Molloy and Julia Serano both say that they spoke with him for the piece, but neither of their contributions made it into the finished article. Indeed, throughout Singal's writing on trans issues, one would be hard-pressed to find many examples of contented trans individuals. Singal often frames his writing in a "just asking questions" perspective, but the frame matters. Around 4 percent of people come to regret having LASIK eye surgery,[11] yet if I wrote an article seeking to understand why people might undergo such surgery and what the lasting effects are but only consulted people from that 4 percent pool of regrets, no amount of statistical asides could undo the felt impact of those personal narratives. It's simply how our brains work. The surgical regret rate for gender confirmation surgery is lower than 4 percent, usually found to be between 1 and 2 percent,[12] yet nearly every article on trans people, particularly trans children, is dominated by this "what if."

Questions have consequences. Seven states cited Singal's writing in a suit to overturn sex discrimination protections for trans people: "By contrast, there is no broad consensus—much less federal law—on the proper approach to treating individuals with gender dysphoria, the clinical term for the feeling of disconnect between one's gender identity and sex at birth. *See, e.g.,* Jesse Singal, *When Children Say They're Trans* . . . (describing the 'growing number of people' who regret transitioning to a different sex and later detransition)."[13] Yet to hear Singal and other gender-critical voices tell it, they are the ones under attack.

While I was writing this chapter, Singal signed onto an open letter alongside noted transphobe J. K. Rowling and others called "A Letter on Justice and Open Debate" and published by *Harper's* in the United States and elsewhere abroad. The letter claims, "The free exchange of information and ideas, the lifeblood of a liberal society, is daily becoming more constricted. While we have come to expect this on the radical right, censoriousness is also spreading more widely in our culture: an intolerance of opposing views, a vogue for public shaming and ostracism, and the tendency to dissolve complex policy issues in a blinding moral certainty."[14] This is, of course, what is so often claimed about trans people and their advocates, that they are blinded by the lights of personal experience and cannot take adequate stock of the scientific evidence. After criticism of the open letter mounted, particularly in light of Singal, Rowling, and other trans-critical signatories, the writer Jennifer Finney Boylan, who is herself transgender, tweeted her regret for signing it, stating on July 7, 2020, "I thought I was endorsing a well meaning, if vague, message against internet shaming." The next day, Rowling tweeted back, "You're still following me, Jennifer. Be sure to publicly repent of your association with Goody Rowling before unfollowing and volunteer to operate the ducking stool next time, as penance," a rather curious reaction if the consideration at hand truly is "free speech."

Humans struggle with difference. We shape stereotypes and patterns of behavior that help us navigate an often perplexing and confusing world, but they often fail us by reducing the full humanity of others to a dull set of characteristics. When faced with difference, whether in regard to who someone finds sexually attractive or how someone conceives of their gender, we have often fallen back onto the well-worn belief that the problem is them. Psychology does not exist above and beyond our prejudices, no matter how much it aspires to scientific objectivity. It has too often started not with a concern for the mental health of others but rather our own discomfort, and mental illness becomes the label we use to classify that discomfort by reassuring ourselves that "they" are the problem.

But "they" are also "us," of course. There are trans mental health professionals just like there were gay mental health professionals back when homosexuality was pathologized. Our understanding of gender and sexuality has grown significantly in just the past few decades, but our diagnoses and our nomenclature have proven slow to catch up. This is a matter not just of proper labeling but of justice; as long as gender dysphoria remains, trans people can still be diagnosed with a mental illness if some facet of them is uncomfortable with being trans, not a difficult task to accomplish in a still-transphobic world. This can impact their ability to be parents, to work the jobs they want, to work at all, to be housed, to be protected from discrimination. Gender dysphoria as a diagnosis is an improvement over gender identity disorder, but it is far from perfect, and it continues to give ammunition to the Rowlings and Singals of the world. Hopefully, in due time their arguments will appear as irrational and off-base as the belief that men became gay because their mothers loved them too much.

Gender and sexuality are not the only arenas in which psychology has struggled to keep up with the surrounding culture. The twentieth century was the most murderous in our recorded history, and all that violence left its mark not only through the dead and injured but those who survived seemingly unscathed.

CHAPTER 5
NO PEACE

For a few years, I was responsible for interviewing aspiring interns at my clinic. Most of them were in the second year of their social work or counseling programs and looking for the opportunity to hone skills learned in the classroom with real patients. The interviewing was mutual; they were also curious about what their time at our clinic might look like and how it might help (or not help) fulfill their professional goals. I cannot claim to be naturally good at this sort of thing, but over time I developed a list of questions that helped me better understand whether or not the person in front of me might be a good match. I would ask about positive experiences they had had in prior internships, about ones that didn't go so smoothly, or about how they might theoretically react to a crisis situation. Once we had established a fairly steady rhythm and they had grown comfortable, I would ask them something that I made sure to ask every candidate who sat in front of me: "How comfortable do you feel working with trauma?"

Some would mishear me and think I was inquiring about their own trauma histories, something I quickly reassured them was none of my business. Most, though, would thoughtfully consider it and, if they did not have experience in a prior role working with trauma survivors (most did not, and I did not expect them to), would say something like, "I haven't really worked with that population yet, but it is something I'm interested in and I really want to learn." This answer did not give me much, but then again, the question wasn't that great either. I always found it difficult to word such questions well, and I attempted to thread the needle between giving them a realistic appraisal of the reality they might face while not scaring them away.

If I were more honest, I would have told them that in the nine months at our clinic, they would almost certainly hear stories of loved ones lost to gun violence. They would work with people who witnessed murders, some who had survived being shot and still carried the scars. They would hear of intimate partner violence, of patients who desperately wanted to escape but felt like they had nowhere to go. They would work with others whose roommates were active drug users and invited other drug users into the home, but their patients would not be able to afford to move. Many of their patients would not feel comfortable leaving their homes, making many of the coping skills the applicants learned in school for depression and anxiety obsolete. They would be more than the sum total of their trauma, of course, but hearing the magnitude of pain they had experienced could easily become overwhelming.

Consider one of my former patients, a Black woman in her fifties named Beverly. Beverly's father was killed by the police when she was a child, allegedly for brandishing a weapon, although this detail was unclear. Beverly's mother became emotionally remote after her husband's death, and Beverly ended up pregnant during high school, which caused her to drop out. Like many other desperate people of her era, she became addicted to crack cocaine. She had two more children, all three of them girls, who were raised by her mother. When they were all teens, she became sober and maintained her sobriety. She had a fractured relationship with each of them, and while she knew why, it caused her no end of grief and sadness. She could not work due to both her mental illness and a host of physical ailments, and even if she had wanted to, there were few jobs in her area. She lived in a neighborhood in which she did not feel safe. In the course of a few months, she witnessed the same drug-dealing teen shot outside her front door three times. She lived with a roommate who was a former romantic partner but whom she could not stand once he began using heroin. She wanted to move but struggled to save anything from her monthly disability check, which was around $700. At one point, she had managed to accrue almost $1,500 and was looking at places, but when one of her daughters told her she was at risk of becoming homeless with her newborn, she gave all of it to her. When we stopped working together, she had begun to save again and hoped that one of her daughters would let her move in with her, although it did not seem like this option was likely to happen.

I use the diagnosis of post-traumatic stress disorder infrequently in my private practice now, but in community mental health, it was one of the most common conditions I saw. We as a society, both mental health professionals and the wider public, have become much more trauma-informed over the last few years. When I was in grad school, there was only one seminar offered on trauma, capped at a handful of students, and only offered twice during my tenure. Even though I knew I desperately needed to become more conversant in the subject, I was never able to get admitted to the seminar. The number of trauma-informed classes have since swelled, and I have noticed the increasing trauma literacy amongst the students I teach.

Within the scope of the *DSM*, the diagnosis of post-traumatic stress disorder is fairly recent. First arriving in 1980, if it were a person it would straddle the divide between Generation X and millennials. Compared to other diagnoses that are composed of a straightforward list of symptoms and a required duration, the criteria for post-traumatic stress disorder are quite complex. In order to qualify for the diagnosis, one must have experienced "actual or threatened death, serious injury, or sexual violence" directly, witnessed it firsthand, or heard about it impacting a loved one; experienced intrusive flashbacks or nightmares of the event; made efforts to avoid triggers for provoking such intrusive memories; experienced changes in memory or mood; have an altered sense of reactivity or arousal (e.g., outbursts of anger, exaggerated startle response); and experienced such symptoms for a period of at least one month. Prior to the creation of the diagnosis in 1980, a person who had experienced a traumatic event would most likely be diagnosed with gross stress reaction (*DSM I*) or transient situational disturbance (*DSM II*), both meant to address the immediate aftermath of the trauma. If a person continued exhibiting symptoms, they required a different diagnosis, communicating an unspoken belief that the inability to quickly "get over" a traumatic event was in itself a sign of mental illness. The fifth edition of the *DSM* moved PTSD from the anxiety disorder section into its own category, thus marking the fact that trauma impacts the individual in a manner different from the trajectory of other forms of mental suffering.

The diagnosis of PTSD has unquestionably evolved in a better direction over the past forty years, yet it fails to capture the reality of many of those patients I used to care for on the West Side of Chicago. The current criteria of PTSD work under the assumption that one has a relatively stable and harmonious picture of the world that is shattered by a horrific event: a car crash, a sexual assault, the murder of a loved one. The resulting symptoms are the result of this schema being violently ripped apart: nightmares and flashbacks, changes in mood, becoming angry or jumpy, and so forth. They fail to fully capture the reality for those that never had such a rosy view of the world in the first place, however.

I mention the life story of Beverly not because it is uniquely sad but because it is so typical of many of the patients I encountered in community mental health. The 2020 murder of George Floyd at the hands of police helped ignite a nationwide conversation on the ways in which white supremacy has structured many of our institutions and core beliefs, but this work is far from over. Beverly lived in communities that experienced deep disinvestment all of her life, had reduced access to good healthcare, had few amenities within walking distance of her apartment (she would not have felt comfortable walking there even if such amenities did exist), and had few options for affordable housing. Which one of these factors, which one of those events I listed above, traumatized her? The answer, of course, is "all of the above," but what is the diagnosis for that?

There have been periodic attempts to widen our understanding of PTSD, usually by creating a second diagnosis to better capture patients like Beverly. Judith Herman, whose book *Trauma and Recovery* (1992) is a milestone in the field of traumatology and who has exerted significant influence on my own work, proposed "complex post-traumatic stress disorder" as a more apt diagnosis for a certain subset of patients. The criteria that Herman outlines include prolonged exposure to trauma over a period of months or years, alterations in affect regulation, alterations in consciousness, alterations in self-perception, alterations in perception of perpetrator(s), alterations in relationships with others, and alterations in systems of meaning.[1] Herman and her colleagues attempted to include the concept, this time under the name "disorders of extreme stress not otherwise specified," in the 1994 *DSM IV* but were rejected due to a purported lack of evidence. In preparation for *DSM 5*, the focus was shifted from adults to children and adolescents and renamed developmental trauma disorder. Again, the diagnosis was rejected.

Outside of the American context of the *DSM*, the idea of complex trauma has gained some traction. In the eleventh revision of the International Classification of Diseases (ICD-11), a guide published by the World Health Organization in 2019, complex post-traumatic stress disorder is included alongside PTSD. The criteria for PTSD are streamlined to just three: re-experiencing the traumatic event, often accompanied by changes in emotion; avoidance of thoughts, memories, activities, or persons that trigger such memories; and persistent perceptions of heightened current threat. Complex PTSD requires those three conditions to be met and establishes three further symptoms: problems in affect regulation, negative thoughts about self or others accompanied by guilt or shame, and difficulties sustaining relationships and feeling close to others. Efforts are made to keep the *DSM* and ICD in alignment, so it remains possible that C-PTSD or something like it will end up in the *DSM* as well.

To understand why the mental health community continues to struggle with the idea that persistent trauma can shatter one's world beyond the already awful experience of the PTSD diagnosis as it stands, it helps to know something about the history of trauma and mental health. War and violence appear in the earliest stories humankind has told itself, sadly ensuring that the condition we now know as PTSD has haunted us for centuries. The modern understanding of trauma, however, is usually traced back to World War I.[2] Traces of it linger in earlier conditions such as hysteria or "railway spine,"[3] a combination of physical and psychological symptoms observed in survivors of train crashes in the second half of the nineteenth century, but it was not until the First World War that observers began to think that external horrific events could trigger internal psychological suffering independent of any organic cause. Even this realization was slow in coming.

It's easy to overlook World War I, especially for Americans whose participation in the conflict was relatively brief. In just four years, an estimated nine million combatants and thirteen million civilians died, chemical weapons and tanks were widely used for the first time, and large swaths of Europe were scarred by trenches. The psychological toll was profound: soldiers screamed and wept, became catatonic, lost their memory and their ability to feel emotion, were plagued by nightmares, had trouble seeing and hearing. The original diagnosis for this condition was "shell shock," believed to be caused by the concussive impact of artillery fire. Physical examinations, however, revealed no somatic cause for this form of suffering. As in earlier debates regarding hysteria and women, the discussion then turned toward the moral character of the soldier.

Some medical professionals took a harsh view toward these patients, believing their symptoms to be a cowardly attempt to avoid serving their country. British psychiatrist Lewis Yealland believed that those with "war neurosis" shared three characteristics in common: weakness of the will, suggestibility, and negativism (being resistant to the idea of recovering). Yealland was authoritarian in his approach, telling patients "If you recover quickly, then it is due to a disease, if you recover slowly, . . . then I shall decide that your condition is due to malingering." He was also liberal in his usage of electric shock, not an uncommon approach in his time but barbaric nonetheless.[4] There were dissenting voices at the time; W. H.R. Rivers practiced a mixture of psychoeducation and talk therapy with his patients, among them the poets Siegfried Sassoon and Robert Graves. Sassoon would later eulogize Rivers in his poem "Revisitation," ending with the line, "And his life's work, in me and many, unfinished."

That "many," however, did not include the vast majority of soldiers who experienced shell shock. Rivers's treatment worked, but it took time; most barely had their suffering acknowledged. Those who were evacuated to the UK to be treated had an understandable reluctance to return to the battlefield, so the preferred treatment by far was brief and as near the front as possible.

In time, the war ended and veterans returned home to a civilian world that did not want to confront the horrors waged on foreign shores. Many suppressed their trauma, and those who could not were placed out of sight in long-term care facilities. As the memory of the war faded, so did the psychological interest in trauma, but in just a few decades, the topic would rise again with the onset of World War II. Some of the earlier progress was retained; psychological responses to trauma were by and large not seen as a moral failure, and it was generally recognized that anyone could experience such symptoms. Multiple researchers found that the greater protection against post-traumatic symptoms were strong bonds with other soldiers in one's unit, so the focus of treatment was providing brief interventions as close to the front lines as possible in order to quickly return the soldier to his support network. This seemed to have worked, at least in terms of the number of soldiers returned to the front line, but little attention was paid to the lasting psychological scars such horrors can leave. The only measure of success at the time was maintaining the ranks, and while the treatment succeeded in that regard, the humanity of the soldiers was lost along the way. They also returned, and like before, they were encouraged to not talk about what they had seen and the topic of trauma faded from memory.

The Vietnam War proved to be different. Far longer than most other conflicts to that point, veterans were able to return to the United States and testify to what they had witnessed while the conflict was ongoing. While small in number, they played a large role in the anti-war movement by providing firsthand knowledge of the sheer terror they experienced. Through their activism, they found community with one another, and the silence that usually descended upon their predecessors was lifted as they realized their suffering was similar. Their work pressured the Veteran's Administration to offer appropriate treatments and spurred further study on the impact of trauma, directly contributing to the formation of the diagnosis of post-traumatic stress disorder.

Alongside these developments, a new wave of feminism was taking shape that bore some similarities to the anti-war movement. Like Vietnam veterans, women began to speak and organize for change, and together they confronted the pervasive nature of sexual trauma and abuse. What was previously seen as a matter of the home became an issue of public concern, leading laws against sexual assault to become far more inclusive throughout the country. Feminists challenged the traditional patriarchal notion that rape was a crime of passion, framing it instead as an act of violence and power. This growing understanding of the psychological impact of sexual assault also helped shape the PTSD diagnosis.

That is largely where we stand at present. Few would argue that we don't need the diagnosis as it stands, but is it really expansive enough to include all that we now call trauma? Even those situations that mostly fit the current standards, such as sexual assault or wartime experiences, are characterized as relatively isolated incidents. The criteria as they stand are not roomy enough to account for all of the other factors that influence how such events are perceived. While allowing for a wide expression of traumatic stress, what "counts" as a traumatic event is rather circumscribed.

Most of us find it difficult to acknowledge, much less attempt to treat, trauma. I cannot count the number of trauma survivors who have told me that, while the trauma itself was horrific, the responses from those around them compounded their pain. Refusing to believe their stories could be true, minimizing their impact or severity, allowing the perpetrator to go unpunished, and/or forcing the survivor to forgive them—these things happen not infrequently. You can witness this happen in real time when a public figure is accused of sexual assault or other misconduct—log on to your social media of choice and see the nauseating takes mount. Survivors see those responses too, and they often serve to churn the leftover memories and scars into a fresh batch of pain.

I would also argue that the current criteria for post-traumatic stress disorder and the unwillingness on the part of the APA to consider a diagnosis of complex trauma contribute to this erasure. In tightening the criteria for PTSD to an event, however painful, considered out of context, we trace psychic pain to an incident in the past rather than a confluence of factors. Being mugged is no doubt horrible for everyone, but it makes a world of difference whether or not the event feels isolated to the survivor, an aberration in an otherwise safe community, or if it seems to confirm every feeling you've had that the neighborhood is unsafe or is the latest in a string of such incidents. A client with experiences like Beverly could undergo the same situation as someone like myself, but the way that we would make sense of it and the support we would receive from those around us would be deeply personal. We maintain a singular focus upon the individual, thereby communicating that other elements of the client's experience do not contribute to the clinical picture.

To consider these factors, or what makes trauma complex, forces us to ask questions beyond the four walls of the therapy room. Violence can happen to anyone, but there are communities in which such events are far more likely to occur. We still find ways to blame the survivors; the summer of 2020 saw a tragic number of children murdered in Chicago, yet the public discourse from the police and other elected officials, after a token expression of sympathy, focuses upon encouraging residents who may have information on the suspects to ignore the prohibitions against snitching and come forward. Communities already mourning a horrific loss are backhandedly blamed for letting the murderers go free while many of the socioeconomic conditions that have contributed to the outbreak of violence are left unexamined. To do that would require us to ask painful questions of ourselves, so instead we assign blame.

In actuality, we are not very far removed from the days of shell shock. We continue to ignore trauma when we can and find ways to blame the survivors when that fails. It took the perfect storm of the Vietnam War and second-wave feminism to finally land PTSD in the pages of the *DSM,* but the diagnosis as it stands maintains a studied determination to be as limited as possible. The same dynamic can be observed when it comes to therapeutic approaches to PTSD.

In 2017 the American Psychological Association published the *Clinical Practice Guideline for the Treatment of Posttraumatic Stress Disorder*, which was meant to be a resource in summarizing the best evidence-based approaches to treating trauma. All of the recommended treatments were based upon randomized controlled trials (RCTs), a hallmark of medicine but something that gets noticeably trickier when applied to therapy. Briefly, RCTs almost always favor manualized, branded forms of therapy because they are believed to provide relatively the same effect despite the therapeutic behavior of the researcher. Further, they are almost always tightly focused; it can be hard enough to find funding for research, so the types of interventions studied are almost always brief, and little follow-up is conducted afterwards. Finally, there isn't unilateral agreement regarding a therapeutic placebo—there are no "sugar pill" talk therapies.[5] It's fine that the *Guideline* included evidence from RCTs, but the exclusive focus upon them predetermines the results.

When therapeutic modalities are tested in such a way, the usual indication that an approach is working is a reduction in symptoms. If you were participating in such a study, you would be given a scale that assigned a number value to your symptoms and their impact upon your life before you began and then would revisit the scale periodically throughout the treatment. This is probably easiest to judge if you are holding a particular incident in mind. In the *This American Life* episode "Ten Sessions," writer Jamie Lowe records the eponymous sessions of a manualized trauma treatment known as Cognitive Processing Therapy (CPT). Lowe experienced a sexual assault as an adolescent and continued to experience some trauma-related symptoms that were further exacerbated by the increased presence of sexual assault in the news. Over a two-week period, she completed an intensive course of CPT, assigning numeric values to various feelings and beliefs and filling out copious worksheets. According to her estimation, it worked: "I don't feel as hopeless and incapacitated when I hear about other assaults. The news doesn't dictate my emotional state in the same way. When Jeffrey Epstein was found dead, I was angry on behalf of his victims. I shouted a few expletives and threw my phone on the ground, but I could still function. And really, that's a very rational reaction."[6]

I agree. And I am glad that Lowe and others are able to find healing and hope without spending years in therapy. But that's not everyone. Most of Lowe's treatment revolves around poking holes in the logical traps she has sewn that keep her suffering: she should not have talked to him that day, she should have worn another outfit, she should have fought back, and so forth. In a case like Lowe's, that works; if the trauma is a history of violence like Beverly's, the logical deductions appear much less clear. She probably is not safe to walk outside at night; her roommate probably does pose a threat to her.

I believe that CPT can work perfectly fine for some of those with PTSD, but I grow concerned when it is presented in such glowing terms as Ira Glass presents it in his introduction to Lowe's story: "There's this kind of therapy for trauma, victims of sexual assault, soldiers with PTSD, where instead of taking years and talking, and talking, and talking on some couch to a therapist with no end in sight, you basically knock it out, all the treatment in just ten or twelve sessions. Two weeks—you can do it in two weeks. And it's effective. Studies have shown that. This therapy's been around since the eighties, but I think lots of people who might find it useful don't even know it's an option for them." The implication here is that long-term, dynamic therapies to address trauma are spinning the patient's wheels when they could find peace much more quickly. I find this troubling whether it occurs professionally in the APA's *Guideline* or in popular media like *This American Life*. Patients can hear it and wonder why they haven't gotten better more quickly. Insurance companies can hear it and wonder why they would pay for anything more than twelve sessions for the diagnostic code of PTSD.

Recovering from trauma is indeed possible, albeit often painful. Throughout history we have often tried to ignore this, instead favoring quick approaches designed to return us to "normality" as quickly as possible, whether that is for soldiers on the front lines or everyday people going about their lives as best they can. If this works, great. But when it often doesn't, that is no mark of failure or shame for the survivor. The dialogue surrounding trauma retains a moralistic quality that has been present from the beginning. The creation of a complex PTSD diagnosis is only a start, but it would be a welcome step in the direction of acknowledging the interlacing factors that can cause so much suffering.

Diagnoses become more muddled the more intervening variables and outside factors we attempt to consider. One of the clearest examples of this is the way the mental health field has tried to talk about intelligence, particularly the purported lack of it.

CHAPTER 6
TIPPING THE SCALES

One of the hardest skills to learn as a beginning therapist is how to work with silence. We know that the work of therapy can be slow, yet when you find yourself sitting across from a person in obvious pain, it can be hard to remember this. Nearly every intern I have supervised tells me within the first few months, "I don't think I'm doing enough. I'm worried I'm going too slow." I would remind them, and myself when needed, that there is no way to speed up the process of developing a relationship, and therapy is premised upon a bond between two people before it is anything else.

Despite knowing this, I faced patients who tested my resolve. One such patient was a young Black woman in her twenties named Sarah. Sarah had been earlier diagnosed with depression and a mild intellectual disability, and her depression was the sort that caused her self-care to decline to the point where she had to be hospitalized upon several occasions in the past. She lived with her mother. She had not graduated high school and did not or could not work. She spent most of her days aimlessly surfing the internet or watching television. Her mother was feeling fed-up, and since she was already a patient at our clinic, she insisted that Sarah start seeing someone as well.

I gleaned all of the above information from Sarah's intake paperwork, but it was not easy. Usually exhaustive and filled with detail, her paperwork was terse, limited. Once I met Sarah, I understood why. She only made eye contact briefly, usually feeling more comfortable to focus her gaze upon the floor. She would answer my questions with one- or two-word answers, even when I carefully sculpted them to elicit more details from her. She was guarded but at the same time fairly open about tensions with her mother. Most patients find silence uncomfortable and work to fill it if the therapist can control their own urge to speak; Sarah let it stretch on for several minutes until I would interject something so I would be able to write down something in my progress notes other than "sat there together."

After quite a few sessions of this with little improvement, I gently broached the idea of change to Sarah. "I don't feel like I'm making you feel comfortable, and I'm wondering if it would be better if I connected you with one of my female coworkers, or at least someone who wasn't a white guy."

"No, I don't want to do that. I feel comfortable with you."

"That's great. I really enjoy meeting together too, but I just want what's best for you. I don't know if I'm helping you. I don't want to make you keep coming here if you're not getting anything from it."

Her eyes snapped up from the floor. "No, you can't do that. No, please."

"Okay, okay, that's fine. What makes you say that though?"

"My mom. She'll kick me out if I don't keep seeing you."

I had some interactions with Sarah's mother as we scheduled her follow-up appointments. She was in many ways the polar opposite of Sarah: telling me the details of her medical travails in the packed waiting room, rolling her eyes in her daughter's direction, asking me how many words I had managed to wrangle out of her each session. I didn't think she would kick Sarah out if we stopped meeting together, but I couldn't be sure of it and didn't want to find out. So we kept our appointments for the next two years until Sarah moved with her mother back to their home state in the Deep South.

Upon reflection, I cannot be sure how Sarah's intellectual disability and depression interacted, how exactly they mixed together to form the shape of her suffering. In settings such as community mental health, a diagnosis of intellectual disability is often a hunch or an observation more than a certainty. If a patient has not been diagnosed while in school when such tests are often available, it is usually quite expensive to have psychological testing done as an adult. Speaking from my own experience, it can be almost impossible to locate a tester who will accept Medicaid or other public insurances.

According to the standards of the *DSM 5*, a diagnosis of intellectual disability requires the onset of intellectual and adaptive deficits during a child's development, and the severity of the disability is measured by the child's performance across the conceptual, social, and practical domains. Alongside these dimensional measures, the child must also have an IQ score two standard deviations below the population mean. The average IQ score is 100, meaning anyone with a score of 70 or below meets the criteria for the diagnosis. I didn't have an IQ score handy for Sarah, but broadly speaking this picture seemed to fit her condition.

IQ tests are not a common feature of community mental health, but in other settings, such as schools, they are ubiquitous. There is strong evidence to suggest that our blind confidence in such measures is misplaced, to say the least. If Sarah had grown up in California, it would have been illegal for her school to administer an IQ test; IQ tests for Black children to determine whether or not they belong in special education were banned there following the 1979 *Larry P.* case.[1] The judge in that case, Robert Peckham, found that Black children were overrepresented in what was then known as educable mentally retarded classes in the San Francisco school district and that the IQ test demonstrated a Eurocentric bias. To date, California remains the only state with such a ruling.

IQ tests don't go away once you leave school, however. They become less formal to be sure but no less intrusive. I often helped clients apply for jobs when they asked. The last few jobs I have personally applied for asked for little more than a cover letter and resume, but I have found that the more low-paying and menial the job, the more hoops required in order to apply. Nearly every big box retail store my clients would apply to required them to complete a battery of questions regarding their responses to stressors they might experience as well as questions that seemed to assess their general knowledge. These questions are merely IQ tests in a different guise.

One might think the *Larry P.* case would be a watershed, but instead it appears to be an outlier. IQ tests continue to dominate our educational system, the labor market, and what gets defined as an intellectual disability. Even when they have not been formally administered, in the case of Sarah or applicants to Target or Walmart, the assumption of an IQ score dictates how one is treated and the sort of opportunities available. How did this one idea come to attain so much significance, and what exactly is it that it's supposed to measure?

The seeds for the modern idea of testing one's intelligence were first sewn in France as the nineteenth century gave way to the twentieth. The then-recent shift to universal public schooling had made it clear to authorities in the Ministry of Education that not all children performed equally well. The ministry turned to a former student of Charcot, Alfred Binet, who was the director of the Laboratory of Physiological Psychology at the Sorbonne. After extensive trial and error, Binet and his assistant, Theodore Simon, developed a series of tests grouped by age that would help determine the mental age of a student. Binet believed that what we call intelligence involved a number of interrelated but separate faculties: attention, memory, common sense, and the like. If a six-year-old got an average number of questions right or wrong on the six-year-old test, they would score 100 and have the mental age of a six-year-old; if they failed to do this, they were assigned a mental age lower than their chronological age and singled out for special attention. Binet intended nothing more for his test than to determine where a particular child at a particular time fell in terms of their academic ability; as he later wrote in his *Les idées modernes sur les enfants* (1909), "Some recent philosophers seem to have given their moral approval to these deplorable verdicts that affirm that the intelligence of an individual is a fixed quantity, a quantity that cannot be augmented. We must protest and react against this brutal pessimism; we will try to demonstrate that it is founded on nothing."

Across the channel in England, another psychiatrist was examining the impact of intelligence on schooling at the same time as Binet. Unlike Binet, Charles Spearman did not think that intelligence was based upon a constellation of faculties but rather could be measured singularly. To prove his point, Spearman examined young children in a village school and found that success in one course was highly correlated with success in all the other courses: a child who did well in French was highly likely to also do well in math and music. Spearman cited this as proof for his theory of general intelligence, or *g*. This represented one half of his two-factor theory of intelligence. As he later wrote, "the measure of every different ability of any person can be resolved into two factors, of which the one is always the same, but the other always independent."[2] So when a child takes a math test, for instance, they utilize the specific skills they have learned about math but are also guided by a general level of intellect that undergirds all of their mental activity. Spearman also believed that no matter the level of *g* one possessed, one's situation-specific skills could make one gifted at a given activity. As he explained it, "Every normal man, woman, and child is, then, a genius at something as well as an idiot at something."

Despite Spearman's cautions, the idea that each person has a measurable quantity of overall intelligence spread rapidly. Binet was interested in measuring intelligence as it corresponded to a child's ability to perform age-specific tasks, and despite the Pandora's box of sorts he opened, his only goal was to determine the mental age of a child. He did not view this as a fixed quantity or statistic but rather as a time-bound marker of one's educational attainment to date. The sort of "brutal pessimism" he warned against, thanks to Spearman's *g*, began to take root.

In the summer of 1908, Henry Herbert Goddard traveled to Europe from the United States to learn the new methods of evaluation Binet had developed. He had recently joined the Vineland Training School for Feeble-Minded Girls and Boys as the director of research and been tasked with making a psychological study of the children there. It only took him a few months to translate the Binet-Simon test into English, and he quickly became its evangelist. American physicians proved eager to adapt the test. By 1913, it was being used to test immigrants at Ellis Island. One year later, Goddard was the first to introduce its findings into a court of law. In the midst of these developments, he published what was to be his most popular book, *The Kallikak Family: A Study in the Heredity of Feeble-Mindedness* (1912).

Goddard claimed that his case study of the Kallikak family came about by investigating the genealogy of one of his patients, Deborah Kallikak. Deborah's great-great-great grandfather, Martin, was a soldier in the Revolutionary War who was married to a Quaker woman. On the way back home from battle, Martin had sex with a "feeble-minded" barmaid who became pregnant. Martin returned home to his family and resumed his upright life, and none of the children he had with his wife demonstrated signs of an intellectual disability. The descendants of the barmaid, however, were blighted by poverty, intellectual disability, and alcoholism, leading all the way to Goddard's patient Deborah. *The Kallikak Family* contained photographs that let the reader witness the "degeneracy" firsthand,[3] increasing the impact of Goddard's narrative. Stephen Jay Gould contended that Goddard manipulated the photographs to appear more menacing, and indeed, upon closer inspection, the pictures do appear to be crudely doctored. Researchers questioned Goddard's methods and conclusions even at the time, but that did not stop his book from becoming a hit.

Goddard was also responsible for coining a word now more familiar as a schoolyard taunt: moron. A moron, derived from the Greek word for "dull," had an intellectual disability but not to the same profound degree as did an "idiot" (with an

IQ score of 0 to 25) or an "imbecile" (with an IQ of 26 to 50). A moron with an IQ usually between 51 and 70 was especially dangerous because they were not as visibly disabled as those in the other two categories. This classification system was used not just to assess one's intellect but also one's potential for criminality and/or becoming a burden upon the system. The category of moron contained all manner of social deviants: criminals, the poor, those with substance use disorders, sex workers, and so forth. As we saw earlier with "sluggish schizophrenia," the concept of moron became another diagnostic tool to punish those who deviated from society's norms. Indeed, Goddard's hope in popularizing the notion of the moron was to serve a warning to the general public who was dangerously ignorant of the existence of this class. This warning came with a solution as well, for Goddard was also a committed eugenicist.

The term "eugenics" was coined in 1883 by Francis Galton, a cousin of Darwin who sought to apply the latter's theory of the development of plants and animals to humans, an elaboration Darwin disagreed with. As discussed earlier in reference to neurasthenia, this period in American history saw rapid shifts in the social landscape of the country as industrialization spread. Genetics was a new field of scientific enquiry, the term being first used in the modern sense in 1905. Increasing immigration ignited xenophobic concerns about the fear of the outsider and the need to maintain some essential core of Americanness that have continued into our own era. Eugenics, or "good breeding," was seen as a way to maintain the essential genetic stock of a country.

Eugenicists sought ways to measure and quantify desirable human traits. The idea of general intelligence seemed perfectly suited for this and replaced earlier, cruder methods such as measuring the skulls of criminals.[4] While the eugenics movement seems to have a pronounced conservative bent, the ranks of eugenicists were filled with many significant figures from the Progressive Era who usually couched their concerns in preventing the spread of poverty, disease, and the like. Theodore Roosevelt, Alexander Graham Bell, and John D. Rockefeller Jr. were all eugenicists, for example. Major foundations sponsored eugenics research. The fervor for eugenics began to influence legislation, especially when it came to immigration and the treatment of the "feeble-minded."

If feeble-mindedness was truly hereditary, they reasoned, the best thing for society is to limit their ability to reproduce through sterilization. Indiana was the first state to successfully pass a sterilization bill in 1907; Washington, California, and Connecticut followed in 1909. Virginia did not pass a sterilization law until 1924, and even then they decided to play it safe. On the advice of counsel, the state's mental hospitals decided to defer on taking action until they tested the law in the courts.

On May 2, 1927, the Supreme Court upheld Virginia's law 8-1 in *Buck v. Bell*, giving new fervor to the eugenics movement. While individual states (including Virginia) have since overturned their sterilization statutes, *Buck v. Bell* still stands. It is estimated that about 70,000 people were sterilized in the United States as a result of the ruling. Forced sterilization never went away; nearly 150 women were sterilized while incarcerated in California between 2006 and 2010.[5] The practice, and eugenics as a whole, however, began to fade from public view during World War II.

The ideal person in the eyes of eugenicists was of Nordic or Anglo-Saxon stock, a prejudice that the Nazis happened to share. Hitler was an admirer of America's eugenics practices, writing in *Mein Kampf*: "There is today one state in which at least weak beginnings toward a better conception are noticeable. Of course, it is not our model German Republic, but the American Union, in which an effort is made to consult reason at least partially. By refusing immigration on principle to elements in poor health, by simply excluding certain races from naturalization, it professes in slow beginnings a view that is peculiar to the folkish state concept." In the early years of his ascent to power, Hitler and the Nazi Party cultivated a warm relationship with American eugenicists. The Rockefeller Foundation donated millions of dollars throughout the 1920s to fund German eugenicists. Unlike in America, where eugenicists were divided up into various camps and organizations, Germany had a single monolithic group, the German Society for Racial Hygiene, which allowed them to accelerate their plans easily. Upon returning to America from Germany in 1934 at a time when the Germans were performing over 5,000 sterilizations a month, the eugenicist C. M. Goethe remarked to a colleague, "You will be interested to know that your work has played a powerful part in shaping the opinions of the group of intellectuals who are behind Hitler in this epoch-making program. Everywhere I sensed that their opinions have been tremendously stimulated by American thought. . . . I want you, my dear friend, to carry this thought with you for the rest of your life, that you have really jolted into action a great government of 60 million people."[6] Once the war started, American fervor for the Nazi's program diminished, at least publicly, as they continued to escalate their program. It is estimated that by the war's end, they had sterilized over 400,000 people and murdered at least 300,000 residents of psychiatric hospitals, not to mention the millions more "undesirables" who were killed in concentration camps. Nazis did not fail to mention the American connection to eugenics in the Nuremberg trials, citing the Supreme Court's decision in the *Buck v. Bell* case in their defense.

Eugenics became much less palatable to the mainstream following the revelations of the Nazi program, yet its ideas lived on in other forms, as did the supposed concern for those with lower IQs. In 1994, the political scientist Charles Murray and the psychologist Richard J. Herrnstein (who died before publication) published their book, *The Bell Curve: Intelligence and Class Structure in American Life*. While the book received a great deal of attention, there was relatively little new about its claims; they utilize Spearman's concept of *g* as their theoretical basis. In examining IQ data according to race, Murray and Herrnstein found that Asian people scored slightly higher than whites while Black people scored significantly lower than both. They claimed that these differences held even when considering a variety of other variables, asserting that these gaps in achievement were genetic in nature. Murray and Herrnstein expressed alarm at the idea that IQ scores across the United States were slipping, blaming them upon increased immigration and the fact that more intelligent people tend to have fewer children than lesser intelligent people. Their suggestion, then, was to limit immigration and eliminate welfare policies that they claim encourage poor women to have more children.

The Bell Curve has been thoroughly debunked, both on its theoretical premises and its conclusions, yet its impact lingers. Charles Murray is distinguished scholar at the American Enterprise Institute, a notable conservative think tank, and continues to publish widely. What is shocking is how much of *The Bell Curve,* despite serious flaws, has become mainstream. While linking IQ to race is widely seen as an example of racist science, in many ways Murray got what he wanted. The same year that his book was released, a Democratic president, Bill Clinton, gutted welfare, and subsequent administrations have continued to hack away at its corpse.

The fear that IQ is dropping in America lingers, even if the quiet part is no longer said out loud. Since the turn of the twenty-first century, IQ scores have demonstrably dropped across Scandinavia, Britain, Germany, France, and Australia. A variety of reasons have been proposed for this, including the rise of less-intellectually demanding jobs, our various devices sapping our ability to focus, or our food becoming less nutritious due to climate change.[7] Lurking behind these theories is the fear that, *Idiocracy*-style, our net intelligence will slip too far, leaving us unable as a society to solve many of the problems that bedevil us.

Perhaps. We should indeed be concerned about the sort of lives technology shapes, the impact of our changing climate upon our food supply, the lack of intellectually stimulating work. I am not sure, though, that IQ is the best framework to discuss these concerns. As we have seen, far too often the notion of an abstract intelligence that can be quantified has been used to justify all manner of evils. It does not seem like too far of a step to assert that, if IQ scores in the United States or elsewhere fell, the actions we would take to "fix" them probably would almost assuredly focus upon those of a lower socioeconomic status or with intellectual disabilities.

This brings us back to the intellectual disability diagnosis. By including dimensional standards for the diagnosis alongside

IQ scores, the *DSM* does begin to right some of the wrongs of our past, but it does not go far enough. While I do not take my ability to reason abstractly for granted, there is nothing about it that makes it fundamentally better than someone else's ability to, say, fix my car. Sarah's life was certainly shaped by her intellectual disability, but what caused her misery was not this but the complete lack of support or understanding she faced at home. I have a relative with an intellectual disability. He is able to live semi-independently in a group home, and he does volunteer work at a local hospital that he takes very seriously. The only thing that makes his work of folding towels less important or meaningful than mine is the standards of our society. The idea that intelligence is something fixed that we can measure will always end up favoring certain expressions of "intelligence" over others, but this is usually based upon their supposed utility to our wider society rather than any intrinsic quality.

We have quite a way to go before people with disabilities, be they intellectual or otherwise, feel included in our society. It is not lost to me that the very same IQ threshold set for a diagnosis of intellectual disability, 70 or lower, continues to follow the moron-imbecile-idiot scale established by Goddard. A diagnosis should be a guide to how we can best help someone, and the IQ test, and the notion of measuring intelligence in general, comes with far too much baggage to be able to do so.

CONCLUSION

I f you ever find yourself in Hollywood but have grown weary of everything showbiz-related, you can always visit the Psychiatry: An Industry of Death museum. Located in the headquarters of its parent organization, the Citizens Commission on Human Rights, one can peruse exhibits that reveal the "real" history of psychiatry that sought to deny the soul and reduced humankind to animality. The Holocaust, racism, Soviet gulags, mind control, school shootings: all are revealed to have been shaped from within by psychiatric practices. Modern psychiatry, the museum contends, has nothing to do with science and is purely profit-driven. The museum also mounts an occasional traveling exhibit, so there's always the possibility of catching it outside of California. Admission is free, but what you won't find at the museum is information on who exactly underwrites its work or that of the Citizens Commission on Human Rights. A quick Google search reveals the answer: the Church of Scientology.

Ever since Tom Cruise jumped on Oprah's couch and accused Matt Lauer of being "glib," the antipsychiatry views of Scientology have been apparent. In offering my own critiques of psychological practice and providing examples of its overreach, I realize I run the risk of aligning myself with those who believe our Earth was populated by the evil galactic emperor Xenu. As I hope has become apparent, I do not think that psychology, at least in the vast majority of cases, is intentionally malicious. Rather, it is something we cannot avoid but often deny. It is human.

There have certainly been actors with bad intentions. Samuel Cartwright was not on the trail of scientific truth when he created drapetomania; he was seeking to ensure the continued subjection of enslaved people. For most, though, concepts and diagnoses both past and present were created to try to help people. The rapid onset of industrialization in America meant that many did indeed struggle to catch up. Women laboring under patriarchy did indeed struggle to get their voices heard and at times resorted to symptoms that seemed strange, even off-putting. This desire to help often included an unspoken belief about how things *should* be: men should want to have sex with women, and soldiers experiencing the horrors of war should want to return to the front lines as soon as possible to help their compatriots.

Psychology is a science, yes, but a peculiar sort of one. Few people are bothered when researchers work to define the healthy functioning of the heart or the liver; it is much harder to suspend judgment when we are trying to define the spectrum of normality for the mind. There is still much we don't understand about how the mind works. Breakthroughs seem to always be around the corner, and indeed our knowledge has grown exponentially in the past few decades compared to ages past. There remains much that is uncharted territory, and I myself am doubtful whether we can ever fully unlock the mysteries contained within.

There is a certain amount of humility that is necessary here, a humility often lacking when it comes to the creation of the disordered. We felt quite certain that Black Americans had no real reasons to resist the various manifestations of white supremacy, so we determined that it was instead an expression of their paranoia. Women had no reason to complain and try to assert their voices against an often-hostile medical establishment, so they must just be hysterical. When we examine the history, these oversights leap out at us, yet we often fail to approach our current formulations with the same amount of skepticism.

It is undoubtedly true that an affliction we now call schizophrenia has existed for centuries and across cultures, yet the way in which we attach meaning to it assigned to race is not inevitable. There is assuredly a segment of the population that struggles with maintaining concentration and attention, yet we far too often fail to examine the ways in which our own lifestyles can contribute to, or even create, these patterns. We do not need to throw out the *DSM* or any other collection of mental suffering, but we do need to be far more modest when it comes to the formulation of what counts as a disorder.

We must also do a better job of taking stock of the social surround of individuals asking for help. All varieties of mental disorders are correlated with external factors that create misery: chronic lack of resources, limited community supports, high levels of violence. I am writing this while under lockdown during the COVID-19 pandemic, and while I have found it stressful, to be sure, I have my own office in which to work, access to necessary resources, and a job that has not gone away but only increased in demand. If any of those factors were different, I might be feeling much worse, yet none of that would be my fault, just like my ability to navigate these times well is not an indicator of some fundamental virtue I possess.

When the Puritans invaded America and stole its land from indigenous peoples, they created a society in which capitalistic production and personal morality were deeply entwined. Few now aspire to the harsh theology of these colonizers, yet this connection, the Protestant work ethic, remains entrenched in our culture. When our production suffers, including through mental illness, it is far too easy for us and others to conclude that we are somehow at fault, the guilty party. This suspicion even lingers within mental health. It is clear that we have much more dismantling to do.

And yet the work continues. There is no lack of people seeking help; in fact, the continued dismantling of these lingering stigmas has reduced the trepidation many experience when they consider mental health treatment. As with everything else connected to healthcare in this country, access is unevenly distributed, but for many the desire is there.

It all starts with listening. When I was in seminary, I found that the internship I was to start in my second year, the internship that I had looked forward to since before I even started my program, no longer appealed to me. In fact, the very idea of starting it filled me with intense anxiety and dread. Not fully understanding why myself, I withdrew and began to consider my options. I had been in therapy briefly before, and it struck me that these were the sort of things that therapy could help. So I went to see a therapist named Ken.

In my work with Ken, we did unearth many of the unconscious dynamics that pushed me toward this decision, but over the years, I also went deeper into myself, achieving a comfort with myself in a way that I never really had before. It made the latter part of my twenties much more enjoyable and fulfilling than the years before. It led me to reconsider an old notion that maybe I would like to do something similar in the future. It made me feel more confident, helped me heal from the pains of a prior relationship, and gave me the courage to send a Facebook message to a friend of a friend who would later become my wife.

The diagnostic code attached to Ken's billing was generalized anxiety disorder, but that doesn't tell my whole story. It isn't even really all that helpful in the end. What Ken and I ended up talking about was, simply, life. No matter what diagnosis gets assigned to us, this is what we all want to work on in the end.

Ken practiced from a client-centered perspective, an approach that is not mine but is similar. He focused on listening, reflecting back what he heard, offering some perspective. At no point did he pull out a manual or send me home with my arms laden with worksheets. That can work sometimes, to be sure, but it largely reduces therapy to a question to be answered rather than a life to be explored. Even when I have adapted such a programmatic approach with a client, I almost always find myself augmenting it with more exploratory questions. If all of life was about utilizing different thought patterns and filling out inventories, we would suffer far less.

All told, I saw Ken over a period of about four years, usually every week but with larger gaps when things were going well. I realize that is often a luxury in our country where insurance company bureaucrats dictate the circumstances of our treatment. I had good enough coverage to allow me to see him at a minimal cost and for a length of time that worked for me. That should be a basic human right when it comes to mental health care, but of course it often does not work out that way.

I do not consider myself "cured" of my anxiety; it still rears its head occasionally, more often recently given the state of the world. I have learned how to relate to it differently, though, and have had my own vision of myself shaped in a way that's far kinder to myself. I hope to be the same sort of force in my clients' lives. When I was in graduate school, there came a definite shift in our coursework where our questions about how therapy might work became less "I've heard that some therapists . . ." and more "I notice that when I say something like that, my therapist responds like this." Nearly all of us had a Ken at some point in our lives.

That is my hope for you as well. We all deserve to have someone listen to our concerns and take them seriously, to really try to understand the shifting dynamics that make up our personalities and do their best to help. At times, diagnoses can help with that, but as I've demonstrated throughout these chapters, far too often that is not the case. The same sort of dynamics can crop up in therapy too; we are not immune from the racism, sexism, transphobia, and so forth of our day. We must try to be better, though, and that starts with a real encounter with the person sitting in front of us.

When I was starting out as a therapist and trying to figure out how to balance all of this, I used to picture placing all of the accrued information I had received regarding a client on the shelf behind my head while I was in session. It was there if I needed it, but it didn't and couldn't get in the way of listening to them. At times, I would find the information confirmed, but often what seemed like a straightforward recitation of symptoms in their intake grew far less clear upon further exploration.

As my understanding of the complicated dynamics and sordid history behind many of our diagnoses grew, I began to place them a little further back on that shelf. They're still there, but I mostly only think about them when I'm doing my billing. Whether my client has schizoaffective disorder or bipolar disorder or depression, my job is pretty much the same. I am there to listen and to try to help. Together we play, and "the play's the thing," to quote Shakespeare. The work continues, always.

ACKNOWLEDGMENTS

I am delighted to be publishing this book with Belt again. I am grateful to Anne Trubek, Martha Bayne, Dan Crissman, and everyone else at Belt who have shepherded my writing along throughout the years, and I'm proud to be a part of our worker-owned, progressive, midwestern publishing family.

In the past few years I have been delighted to teach psychodynamic practice methods to the wonderful students at my alma mater, the University of Chicago School of Social Service Administration (recently renamed the Crown Family of Social Work, Policy, and Practice). While they are too many to name, I am thankful to every one of them for asking penetrating, insightful questions into this particular business of the mind and its functioning while staying ever aware of the social justice work that is our commitment as social workers. I am also grateful to my fellow lecturers in the psychodynamic track, Kevin Barrett and Jennifer Cutilletta, for their insight and care as we have worked together to harmonize our curriculum.

I am also grateful to my coworkers at the Claret Center who have demonstrated boundless enthusiasm for my writing and are always receptive to my works in progress. And I remain ever appreciative to Catherine Ortiz, who gave me my start at Mt. Sinai, as well as all of my colleagues there who played so vital a role in my development. Thanks are also due to everyone at the Chicago Center for Psychoanalysis who have created fertile ground for intellectual exploration for the sake of others. My work has grown immeasurably through my affiliation there.

When I signed the contract for this book early in 2020, I in no way anticipated writing it while quarantined due to a deadly pandemic. In the days of reduced social circles, I grew even more grateful for our family and the myriad ways in which they offered support. While I look forward to the day when our interactions are not facilitated through a computer screen, I felt overwhelmingly supported despite the distance. My parents, Cindy and Duane Askins and Neil and Patty Foiles, always helped keep me encouraged, and my in-laws, Juan and Suzanne Angulo, helped keep me going in the writing when it felt like a slog. The pandemic has also laid bare how unequal childcare in this country can be, so I must acknowledge the invaluable help the Angulos provided in watching our children while my wife and I worked out of our condo.

My friends have been welcome interlocutors through the shaping of this book. I owe a particular debt of thanks to Joe Grant who assured me that the idea for this book is something people might want to read and introduced me to the work of Arnold Davidson, which helped jumpstart my process.

My son, Edmond William, was born six weeks before the release of *This City Is Killing Me*. It made for an interesting book promotion season, although I probably would have been sleepless anyway. He has been on the other side of the door for most of the writing of this, and upon revising the manuscript, I felt like I could watch him grow through the pages. This book is for him. I also cannot forget my wonderful wife, Esther, best of wives and best of women. Without her loving care and attention, for both me and for our children, this book would not have been possible. And, of course, there's our daughter, Elena, who with her brother has been a bright spot beyond recounting during a troubling time. My love and gratitude for each of them is immeasurable.

NOTES

Introduction

1 Jonathan Leo and Jeffrey Lacasse, "The Media and the Chemical Imbalance Theory of Depression," *Society* 45 (2008): 35–45.

2 Original Zoloft Commercial, YouTube, https://www.youtube.com/watch?v=twhvtzd6gXA&list=PL_V67p-zEfTFfSE2NNseE0FFKU1GEHNyT&index=3.

3 Joshua Kemp, James Lickel, and Brett Deacon, "Effects of a Chemical Imbalance Causal Explanation on Individuals' Perceptions of Their Depressive Symptoms," *Behaviour Research and Therapy* 56 (2014): 47–52.

4 Arnold Davidson, *The Emergence of Sexuality: Historical Epistemology and the Formation of Concepts* (Cambridge, MA: Harvard University Press, 2001).

5 Alex Kwong, José Lopéz-Lopéz, Gemma Hammerton, et al., "Genetic and Environmental Risk Factors Associated with Trajectories of Depression Symptoms from Adolescence to Young Adulthood," *JAMA Network Open* 2, no. 6 (2019).

6 Esmé Weijun Wang, *The Collected Schizophrenias* (Minneapolis: Graywolf Press, 2019).

Chapter 1

[1] Jonathan Metzl, *The Protest Psychosis: How Schizophrenia Became a Black Disease* (Boston: Beacon Press, 2011).

[2] Harold Neighbors et al., "Race, Ethnicity, and the Use of Services for Mental Disorders: Results from the National Survey of American Life," *Archives of General Psychiatry* 64, no. 4 (2007): 485–494.

[3] Julie B. Malinger et al., "Racial Disparities in the Use of Second-Generation Antipsychotics for the Treatment of Schizophrenia," *Psychiatric Services* 57, no. 1 (Jan 2006): 133–136.

[4] Eri Kuno and Aileen Rothbard, "Racial Disparities in Antipsychotic Prescription Patterns for Patients with Schizophrenia," *The American Journal of Psychiatry* 159, no. 4 (April 2002): 567–572.

[5] Michele Solis, "Searching for Schizophrenia," *Science History Institute,* November 19, 2019, https://www.sciencehistory.org/distillations/searching-for-schizophrenia.

[6] Walter Bromberg and Franck Simon, "The Protest Psychosis: A Special Type of Reactive Psychosis," *Archives of General Psychiatry* 19, no. 2 (1968): 155–160.

[7] Walter Reich, "The World of Society Psychiatry," *New York Times,* January 30, 1983, https://www.nytimes.com/1983/01/30/magazine/the-world-of-soviet-psychiatry.html.

[8] National Research Council, *The Growth of Incarceration in the United States: Exploring Causes and Consequences* (Washington, DC: The National Academies Press, 2014).

[9] Lorna Collier, "Incarceration Nation," *American Psychological Association*, October 2014, https://www.apa.org/monitor/2014/10/incarceration.

[10] Bob Myers, "'Drapetomania': Rebellion, Defiance, and Free Black Insanity in the Antebellum United States" (PhD diss., University of California, Los Angeles, 2014), eScholarship.

[11] Samuel Cartwright, "Diseases and Particularities of the Negro Race," *De Bow's Review* 11 (1851).

[12] E.g., W. Wolfgang Fleischhacker et al., "Schizophrenia— Time to Commit Policy Change," *Schizophrenia Bulletin* 40, Issue Supplement 3, (April 2014): S165–S194.

Chapter 2

[1] Lisa Weyandt et al., "Prescription Stimulant Misuse: Where Are We and Where Do We Go From Here?" *Experimental and Clinical Psychopharmacology* 24, no. 5 (2016): 400–414.

[2] Rachel Bluth, "ADHD Numbers are Rising, and Scientists are Trying to Understand Why," *Washington Post,* September 10, 2018, https://www.washingtonpost.com/national/health-science/adhd-numbers-are-rising-and-scientists-are-trying-to-understand-why/2018/09/07/a918d0f4-b07e-11e8-a20b-5f4f84429666_story.html.

3 Paul Morgan et al., "Racial and Ethnic Disparities in ADHD Diagnosis from Kindergarten to Eighth Grade," *Pediatrics* 132, no. 1 (2013): 85–93.

4 See, e.g., Faraone, Stephen V et al. "The worldwide prevalence of ADHD: is it an American condition?," *World Psychiatry: Official Journal of the World Psychiatric Association* 2, no. 2 (2003): 104–13.

5 Hannah Sampson, "What Does America Have Against Vacation?" *Washington Post,* August 28, 2019, https://www.washingtonpost.com/travel/2019/08/28/what-does-america-have-against-vacation/.

6 HospitalityNet, "Americans Multitask More than Any Other Country—Suppressing Their Creativity and Inspiration," November 5, 2019, https://www.hospitalitynet.org/news/4095725.html.

7 L. Mark Carrier et al., "Multitasking Across Generations: Multitasking Choices and Difficulty Ratings in Three Generations of Americans," *Computers in Human Behavior* 25, no. 2 (March 2009): 483–489.

8 Jagdish Khubchandani and James Price, "Short Sleep Duration in Working American Adults, 2010–2018," *Journal of Community Health* 45 (2020): 219–227.

9 Derek Thompson, "Workism is Making Americans Miserable," *The Atlantic,* February 24, 2019, https://www.theatlantic.com/ideas/archive/2019/02/religion-workism-making-americans-miserable/583441/.

[10] Economic Policy Institute, "The Productivity-Pay Gap," July 2019, https://www.epi.org/productivity-pay-gap/.

[11] S. Weir Mitchell, *Wear and Tear, or Hints for the Overworked* (Philadelphia: J. B. Lippincott, 1891).

[12] Matthew Fadus et al., "Unconscious Bias and the Diagnosis of Disruptive Behavior Disorders and ADHD in African American and Hispanic Youth," *Academic Psychiatry* 44 (2020): 95–102.

Chapter 3

[1] Akiskal, H. S. et al., "Borderline: An Adjective in Search of a Noun," *The Journal of Clinical Psychiatry* 46, no. 2 (1985): 41–48.

[2] John Gunderson, "Borderline Personality Disorder: Ontogeny of a Diagnosis," *American Journal of Psychiatry* 166, no. 5 (2009): 530–539.

[3] Randy Sansone and Lori A. Sansone, "Gender Patterns in Borderline Personality Disorder," *Innovations in Clinical Neuroscience* 8, no. 5 (2011): 16–20.

[4] Klonsky, E. David et al., "Gender Role and Personality Disorders," *Journal of Personality Disorders* 16, no. 5 (2002): 464–476. Note that the original uses the clumsy and, to my ears, offensive language of "feminine-acting men" and "masculine-acting women." I have updated the terms used to be more in line with acceptable designations for those who do not conform to the gender binary.

[5] Lillebeth Larun and Kirsti Malterud, "Identity and Coping Experiences in Chronic Fatigue Syndrome: A Synthesis of Qualitative Studies," *Patient Education and Counseling* 69, no. 1–3 (2007): 20–28.

[6] Laura Hillenbrand, "A Sudden Illness," *The New Yorker,* June 30, 2003, https://www.newyorker.com/magazine/2003/07/07/a-sudden-illness.

Chapter 4

[1] Jack Drescher, "Queer Diagnoses Revisited: The Past and Future of Homosexuality and Gender Diagnoses in DSM and ICD," *International Review of Psychiatry* 27, no. 5 (2015): 386–95.

[2] Ronald Bayer, *Homosexuality & American Psychiatry: The Politics of Diagnosis* (Princeton, NJ: Princeton University Press, 1987).

[3] Ibid.

[4] Gary Alinder, "Gay Liberation Meets the Shrinks,"in *Out of the Closet: Voices of Gay Liberation*, 2nd ed., ed. Karla Jay and Allen Young (New York: NYU Press, 1992), 141–144.

[5] Alix Spiegel, "81 Words," *This American Life,* podcast audio, January 18, 2002, https://www.thisamericanlife.org/204/81-words.

[6] Anand Satiani et al., "Projected Workforce of Psychiatrists in the United States: A Population Analysis," *Psychiatric Services* 69, no. 6 (June 2018): 710–713.

[7] Julia Serano, "The Case Against Autogynephilia," *International Journal of Transgenderism* 12, no. 3 (2010): 176–187.

[8] Alix Spiegel, "Two Families Grapple with Sons' Gender Identities," *All Things Considered,* May 7, 2008, https://www.npr.org/2008/05/07/90247842/two-families-grapple-with-sons-gender-preferences.

[9] Jesse Singal, "How the Fight Over Transgender Kids Got a Leading Sex Researcher Fired," *The Cut,* February 7, 2016, https://www.thecut.com/2016/02/fight-over-trans-kids-got-a-researcher-fired.html.

[10] Ana Valens, "Journalist Jesse Singal Says He 'Goofed' On Interpreting Trans Study—And Activists Are Infuriated," *Daily Dot,* March 29, 2018, https://www.dailydot.com/irl/jesse-singal-trans-children/.

[11] American Refractive Surgery Council, "LASIK Complication Rate: The Latest Facts and Stats You Should Know," October 30, 2017, https://americanrefractivesurgerycouncil.org/lasik-complication-rate-latest-facts/.

[12] Brynn Tannehill, "Myths About Transition Regrets," *HuffPost,* November 18, 2014, https://www.huffpost.com/entry/myths-about-transition-regrets_b_6160626.

[13] Franciscan Alliance Inc. v. Azar, "Reply Brief in Support of State Plaintiffs' Renewed Motion for Summary Judgment," filed May 3, 2019, https://affordablecareactlitigation.files.wordpress.com/2019/05/state-plaintiffs-sj-reply-5-3-19.pdf.

[14] "A Letter on Justice and Open Debate," *Harper's Magazine,* July 7, 2020, https://harpers.org/a-letter-on-justice-and-open-debate/.

Chapter 5

[1] Judith Herman, *Trauma and Recovery: The Aftermath of Violence—From Domestic Abuse to Political Terror,* rev. ed. (New York: Basic Books, 2015).

[2] For the following history see Herman, *Trauma and Recovery.*

[3] Ralph Harrington, "On the Tracks of Trauma: Railway Spine Reconsidered," *Social History of Medicine* 16, no. 2 (August 2003): 209–223.

[4] Stefanie Linden, Edgar Jones, and Andrew Lees, "Shell Shock at Queen Square: Lewis Yealland 100 Years On," *Brain* 136, no. 6 (June 2013): 1976–1988.

[5] For further critique see V. Barry Dauphin, "A critique of the American Psychological Association Clinical Practice Guideline for the Treatment of Posttraumatic Stress Disorder (PTSD) in Adults," *Psychoanalytic Psychology* 37, no. 2 (2020): 117–127.

[6] Jaime Lowe, "Ten Sessions," *This American Life,* podcast audio, August 23, 2019, https://www.thisamericanlife.org/682/transcript.

Chapter 6

[1] For more on the *Larry P.* case, see Lee Romney, Rachael Cusick, and Pat Walters, "G: The Miseducation of Larry P," *Radiolab,* podcast episode, June 7, 2019, https://www.wnycstudios.org/podcasts/radiolab/articles/g-miseducation-larry-p.

[2] Charles Spearman, "Some Issues in the Theory of 'g' (Including the Law of Diminishing Returns)," *Nature* 116, no. 2916 (September 19, 1925): 436–439.

[3] Evan Chaloupka, "Imagining Cognitive Disability: Recursive Reading and Viewing Processes in Henry H. Goddard's *The Kallikak Family: A Study in the Heredity of Feeblemindedness,"* *CEA Critic* 77, no. 3 (2015): 269–277.

[4] Ajitha Reddy, "The Eugenic Origins of IQ Testing: Implications for Post Atkins Litigation," *DePaul Law Review* 57, no. 3 (2008): 667–678.

[5] Hunter Schwarz, "Following Reports of Forced Sterilization of Female Prison Inmates, California Passes Ban," *The Washington Post,* September 26, 2014, https://www.washingtonpost.com/blogs/govbeat/wp/2014/09/26/following-reports-of-forced-sterilization-of-female-prison-inmates-california-passes-ban/.

[6] Edwin Black, "Eugenics and the Nazis—The California Connection," *SFGate,* November 9, 2003, https://www.sfgate.com/opinion/article/Eugenics-and-the-Nazis-the-California-2549771.php.

[7] Evan Horowitz, "IQ Rates are Dropping in Many Developed Countries and That Doesn't Bode Well for Humanity," *NBC New Think,* May 22, 2019, https://www.nbcnews.com/think/opinion/iq-rates-are-dropping-many-developed-countries-doesn-t-bode-ncna1008576.

CPSIA information can be obtained
at www.ICGtesting.com
Printed in the USA
JSHW040006300721
17291JS00005B/6